CHINESE TUI NA MASSAGE

CHINESE TUI NA MASSAGE

The Essential Guide to Treating Injuries,
Improving Health, & Balancing Qi

XU, XIANGCAI

YMAA Publication Center
Boston, Mass. USA

YMAA Publication Center
Main Office:
    4354 Washington Street
    Boston, Massachusetts, 02131
    617-323-7215 • ymaa@aol.com • www.ymaa.com

POD 1105

Copyright ©2002 by Xu Xiangcai

ISBN:1-886969-04-3

Edited by Sharon Rose
Cover design by Richard Rossiter

Publisher's Cataloging in Publication
(Prepared by Quality Books Inc.)

Xu, Xiangcai.
    Chinese tui na massage : the essential guide to
treating injuries, improving health, & balancing qi / Xu
Xiangcai. — 1nd ed.
    p. cm.
    Includes index.
    LCCN: 2002101836
    ISBN: 1-886969-04-3

    1. Massage therapy. 2. Medicine, Chinese.
I. Title.

RM723.C5X89 2002   615.8'22'0951
                                QBI02-200316

Disclaimer:
    The authors and publisher of this material are NOT RESPONSIBLE in any
manner whatsoever for any injury which may occur through reading or following
the instructions in this manual.
    The activities, physical or otherwise, described in this material may be too
strenuous or dangerous for some people, and the reader(s) should consult a
physician before engaging in them.

Table of Contents

Table of Contents

Editor's Notes

This volume offers information about the following topics:
- An introduction to tuina
- Methods and steps to learn proper structure and performance of tuina manipulations
- Mandatory exercises to practice the manipulations
- Commonly used manipulations for tuina
- Treatments of common adult diseases
- Self-tuina for preventative healthcare

Note: This text focuses on proper execution of tuina techniques and, therefore, assumes you have been trained in necessary diagnostic techniques.

To make the most of this learning experience, follow three easy steps.

1. Make sure you understand the basics of TCM. (This book assumes you have basic knowledge of Western medicine, massage therapy, and/or human anatomy and physiology). The level of your understanding of the basics will determine the level of proficiency that you can achieve in performing tuina. Generally speaking, one can master tuina techniques as long as s/he studies conscientiously and practices hard according to this book. Those with sound basic knowledge of TCM and/or Western medicine will grasp the essentials of tuina much more quickly. However, to perform at the level of a master tuina practitioner and to perform the more technically difficult manipulations with high proficiency (such as those of Yi Zhi Chan Tui Fa and Gun Fa) is impossible unless long-term professional training has been achieved.

2. Follow the directions in the Exercise Training sections of this book. Conscientiously perform the commonly used exercises according to the accepted training methods to adequately improve your own health, strength, and endurance as needed for a tuina specialty.

3. Practice the basic manipulations as described in the Commonly Used Manipulations sections of this book. Always remember the basic movement mechanism and technical essentials of every maneuver. To master the manipulation skills, strictly following the required training methods and procedures, proceed step-by-step, and practice, practice, practice—first on a bag filled with rice and then on the human body.

Foreword

I am delighted to learn that *Chinese Tui Na Massage* will soon come into the world. TCM has experienced many vicissitudes of times but has remained evergreen. It has made great contributions not only to the power and prosperity of our Chinese nation but to the enrichment and improvement of world medicine. Unfortunately, differences in nations, states and languages have slowed down its spreading and flowing outside China. Presently, however, an upsurge in learning, researching and applying Traditional Chinese Medicine (TCM) is unfolding. In order to bring the practice of TCM to all areas of the globe, Mr. Xu Xiangcai called intellectuals of noble aspirations and high intelligence together from Shandong and many other provinces in China to compile and translate this text. I believe that the day when the world's medicine is fully developed will be the day when TCM has spread throughout the world.

I am pleased to give it my recommendation.

Prof. Dr. Hu Ximing

*Deputy Minister of the Ministry of Public Health of
the People's Republic of China, Director General of the
State Administrative Bureau of Traditional Chinese,
Medicine and Pharmacology, President of the World
Federation of Acupuncture Moxibustion Societies, Member
of China Association of Science & Technology, Deputy
President of All-China Association of Traditional
Chinese Medicine, President of China Acupuncture &
Moxibustion Society*

Foreword

The Chinese nation has been through a long, arduous course of struggling against diseases and has developed its own traditional medicine—Traditional Chinese Medicine and Pharmacology (TCMP). TCMP employs a unique, comprehensive, scientific system including both theories and clinical practice. Some thousand years since its beginnings, not only has TCMP been well preserved but also continuously developed. It has special advantages, such as remarkable curative effects and few side effects. Hence, it is an effective means by which people prevent and treat diseases and keep themselves strong and healthy.

All achievements attained by any nation in the development of medicine are the public wealth of all humankind. They should not be confined within a single country. What is more, the need to set them free to flow throughout the world as quickly and precisely as possible is greater than that of any other kind of science. During my more than thirty years of being engaged in Traditional Chinese Medicine (TCM), I have looked forward to the day when TCMP will have spread all over the world and made its contributions to the elimination of diseases of all humankind. However, I deeply regret that the pace of TCMP in extending outside China has been unsatisfactory due to the major difficulties in expressing its concepts in foreign languages.

Mr. Xu Xiangcai, a teacher of Shandong College of Traditional Chinese Medicine, has sponsored and taken charge of the work of compilation and translation of *The English-Chinese Encyclopedia of Practical Traditional Chinese Medicine*—an extensive series. This work is a great project, a large-scale scientific research, a courageous effort and a novel creation. I deeply esteem Mr. Xu Xiangcai and his compilers and translators, who have been working day and night for such a long time. I admire them for their hard labor, for the firm and indomitable will they displayed in overcoming one difficulty after another and for their great success achieved in this way. As a leader in the circles of TCM, I am duty bound to do my best to support them.

I believe this encyclopedia will be certain to find its position both in the history of Chinese medicine and in the history of world science and technology.

Mr. Zhang Qiwen
Member of the Standing Committee of All-China Association of TCM, Deputy Head of the Health Department Shandong Province

Preface

Traditional Chinese Medicine (TCM) is one of China's great cultural heritages. Since the founding of the People's Republic of China in 1949, the treasure house of the theories of TCM has been continuously explored and the plentiful literature researched and compiled. The effort was guided by the farsighted TCM policy of the Chinese Communist Party and the Chinese government. As a result, great success has been achieved. Today, a worldwide upsurge has appeared in the studying and researching of TCM. To promote even more vigorous development of this trend in order that TCM may better serve all humankind, efforts are required to further it throughout the world. To bring this about, the language barriers must be overcome as soon as possible in order that TCM can be accurately expressed in foreign languages. Thus, the compilation and translation of a series of English-Chinese books of basic knowledge of TCM has become of great urgency to serve the needs of medical and educational circles both inside and outside China.

In recent years, at the request of the health departments, satisfactory achievements have been made in researching the expression of TCM in English. Based on the investigation into the history and current state of the research work mentioned above, *The English-Chinese Encyclopedia of Practical Traditional Chinese Medicine* has been published to meet the needs of extending the knowledge of TCM around the world.

The encyclopedia consists of twenty-one volumes, each dealing with a particular branch of TCM. In the process of compilation, the distinguishing features of TCM have been given close attention and great efforts have been made to ensure that the content is scientific, practical, comprehensive and concise. The chief writers of the Chinese manuscripts include professors or associate professors with at least twenty years of practical clinical and/or teaching experience in TCM. The Chinese manuscript of each volume has been checked and approved by a specialist of the relevant branch of TCM. The team of the translators and revisers of the English versions consists of TCM specialists with a good command of English professional medical translators and teachers of English from TCM colleges or universities. At a symposium to standardize the English versions, scholars from twenty-two colleges or universities, research institutes of TCM or other health institutes probed the question of how to express TCM in English more comprehensively, systematically and accurately and discussed and deliberated in detail the

English versions of some volumes in order to upgrade the English versions of the whole series. The English version of each volume has been re-examined and then given a final checking. Obviously this encyclopedia will provide extensive reading material of TCM English for senior students in colleges of TCM in China and will also greatly benefit foreigners studying TCM. The diligent efforts of compiling and translating this encyclopedia have been supported by the responsible leaders of three organizations:

1. State Education Commission of the People's Republic of China

2. State Administrative Bureau of TCM and Pharmacy and the Education Commission

3. Health Department of Shandong Province

Under the direction of the Higher Education Department of the State Education Commission, the leading board of compilation and translation of this encyclopedia was created. The leaders of many colleges of TCM and pharmaceutical factories of TCM have also given assistance.

We hope that this encyclopedia will promote further and improve instruction of TCM in English at the colleges of TCM in China, cultivate the sharing of ideas of TCM in English in medical circles and give impetus to the study of TCM outside China.

CHAPTER 1

Introduction to Tuina

In ancient China, therapy was classified based on how each therapy was administered; it was either external or internal. One external type of therapy is tuina, a branch of medicine guided by the theories of Traditional Chinese Medicine (TCM). TCM is founded on the concepts of treating the body as an integrated whole, the theory of *yin* and *yang*, five element theory, and the meridians—including primary channels, collaterals, and acupoints.

In tuina, manipulations are used to stimulate points or other parts of the body surface to correct physiological imbalance in the body and achieve curative effects. That is, tuina dredges the channels and collaterals, promotes blood circulation, and regulates *yin* and *yang* so as to return body functions to normal.

Since the primary effect of tuina is to restore balance, tuina increases or decreases the body's functions to combat either excess or deficiency as appropriate. For this reason, tuina is said to regulate dual-directionally. For instance, tuina practiced on appropriate points over the abdomen and back (or arms) returns abnormal peristalsis to normal—regardless of whether the patient suffers from *hyper*peristalsis or *hypo*peristalsis.

In general, the effect of tuina is twofold: smoothing and checking. Smoothing means dispersing obstruction, while checking means restraining hyperfunction.

1.1 Tuina as Therapy

Tuina is traditionally and most often used to treat the following:
- Cervical spondylosis
- Lumbar muscle strain
- Acute lumbar muscle sprain
- Prolapse of lumbar intervertebral disc
- Rheumatoid arthritis
- Epigastralgia

- Gastroptosia
- Constipation
- Hypertension
- Apoplexy
- Diabetes

Additionally, allergic colitis and duodenal bulbar ulcers heal more quickly when they are treated with tuina, and, in recent years, tuina treatments of chronic coronary disorders and angina pectoris have been very successful.

1.2 Tuina as Preventive Healthcare

Tuina may be used not only to treat diseases but also to protect health and build up the body to prevent disease. By practicing self-tuina, Chinese forefathers kept their *qi* and blood flowing freely, strengthened their tendons and bones, eliminated fatigue and restlessness, and promoted longevity.

1.3 Tuina History

As seen throughout medical history, people of medicine often use their hands to treat or prevent diseases. In primitive times when there were neither medical instruments nor drugs to treat diseases, our ancestors could do nothing but use the spontaneous medical methods of self-rubbing, self-kneading or pounding, and stepping on each other. They rubbed, pressed, kneaded, or pounded their own or their patients' bodies in order to keep out the cold; warm themselves; and eliminate fatigue, abdominal distention, and various injuries.

This instinct and proven practice is the origin of Tuina. Chinese forefathers organized the practice into a formal therapy and continually developed their practical experiences over time. Gradually, this therapy became what is called now the natural therapy of tuina.

The following are key milestones in tuina's evolution.

The reign of Emperor Huang. Tunia exists as a practice called *anwu*.

Warring Stages (two thousand years ago). Tuina is called *anmo* and develops into a widely used and more organized medical therapy. For example, Bian Que, an outstanding physician living in that time, once used a comprehensive therapy including *anmo* to treat a crown prince of the state of Guo who was suffering from corpse-like syncope. Reportedly *anmo* drew him back from the jaws of death.

The dynasties of Qin and Han. A dissertation on *anmo* entitled *Huang Di Qi Bo An Mo Jing Shi Juan* is written. This is followed by the Chinese medical classic, *Nei Jing*, which contains many chapters dealing with nearly all aspects of *anmo* therapy (the origin, manipulations, clinical application, indications, therapeutic principles and teaching). The experiences obtained and the methods created both in the past medical practice are enriched and summed up step-by-step.

The time of the Three Kingdoms.

- *Gaomo* enhances the practice of *anmo* therapy, by first smearing an ointment made from herbal medicines on the patient's body surface. Zhang Zhongjing advances and summarizes the method of *gaomo* in the book *Jin Kui Yao Lue*.

- Hua Tuo uses this method to treat febrile diseases and get rid of superficial pathogens in the skin, expanding the uses for which *anmo* and *gaomo* are effective.

The time of the West Jin, East Jin and Northern and Southern Dynasties (265-568 A.D.), *gaomo* technique is further developed.

- In the book *Mai Jing*, Wang Shuhe outlines a way in which pain due to arthralgia syndrome is treated with an ointment *fenggao*.

- Ge Hong systematically sums up the prescriptions, drugs, indications, and operations of *gaomo* in the book, *Zhou Hou Bei Ji Fang*.

- Tao Hongjing's book, *Yang Xing Yan Ming Lu*, addresses physical and breathing exercises combined with self-massage aimed at preventative healthcare and self-treatment of diseases.

Dynasties of Sui and Tang.

- *Anmo* is officially set up in the State Office of Imperial Physicians. Massage practitioners fell into different degrees: doctor (referring to one with doctorate), physician, and technician. With the help of physicians and workers, doctors took charge of the medical work and classroom instruction of massage.

- Sun Simiao's book, *Qian Jin Fang*, is the first to discuss the treatment of more than ten infantile diseases with *gaomo* therapy.

- *Anmo*, as a clinical subject of TCM, makes great advances in its system of basic theory, diagnostic technique, and treatment of several diseases in adults and infants.

- The practice of *anmo* spreads to foreign countries such as Korea, Japan, and India. (During this time, the exchange of culture and ideas between China and other countries thrives due to the greater development of politics, economy, culture, and transportation.)

Dynasties of Song, Jin, and Yuan.

- *Anmo* therapy is mainly used to treat disorders or osteotrauma and lays the foundations for the medical system of bone setting with tuina.

- *Anmo* is used to expedite child delivery.

Ming Dynasty. The term *tuina* appears for the first time and indicates the flourish of *anmo* as a distinct academic branch with its own specific system of diagnosis, manipulations and points. (The innovation of subject terminology, i.e., "tuina" is a sign that this subject has been raised to a high level as a whole.)

Qing Dynasty.

- Tuina is frowned upon by the government and yet spreads rather extensively among the people. Remarkable developments are made.

- Methods for treating fractures and trauma are developed and practiced. The medical branch of traumatology using tuina is formed.

After the foundation of the People's Republic of China in 1949.
The government advocates TCM with a great effort and looks at tuina medicine with a new eye.

- In 1956, the first tuina training class is held in Shanghai.

- In 1958, Shanghai Clinic of Tuina and Shanghai Technical Secondary School of Tuina are set up.

- Up to 1960s, a professional contingent of tuina is formed in China. Folk tuina practitioners all over China are assigned to hospitals to work in the clinical departments of tuina.

- In 1974, the first tuina section appears at the department of Acupunture, Tuina and Traumatology in Shanghai College of TCM. Later, the same thing happens in the TCM colleges of Beijing, Nanjing, Fujian and Anhui. This provides conditions for cultivating outstanding tuina physicians.

- In 1987, the All-China Association of Tuina was created. From then on, academic exchanges of Tuina, national or international, are conducted vigorously.

Today. Tuina medicine flourishes in China and plays an active part in various medical fields such as medical service, rehabilitation, and prevention. Its safe, effective, and harmless advantages without side effects are to be known and accepted by the people all over the world.

1.4 Modern Research of Tuina Manipulations

Research as to "why" tuina actually has the effects it does is underway and no real answers exist yet. However, significant information has been gathered as to what factors of manipulations provide the greatest results. To gather information about the dynamic force of manipulation, the causality between a manipulation and the force it produces, and TCM principles' effects of the maneuvers of tuina, the TDL-I Analyzer for Determining the Dynamic Force of Tuina Manipulation was developed. (See Figure 1). and combined it in 1981 with a corresponding secondary meter, Measuring and Recording System of the Mechanical Information of Tuina Manipulation (See Figure 2). In 1984, we combined it with another instrument called the Computer-process System of the Mechanical Information of Tuina Manipulation (See Figure 3). Since then, we continue to perform systematic sports biomechanical researches—with those instruments—on the manipulations of modern academic authorities of different tuina schools. We record tri-dimensional mechanical waviness-curve diagrams of tuina manipulations (See Figures 4, 5, 6, 7, 8), and perform kinematics and dynamics analysis of each manipulation and its diagram. By so doing, we obtain the objective quantitative index of the experience and technical secrets of tuina manipulation, which previously could only be realized through one's own experience (not be learned from a teacher). Now these secrets may begin to be expressed in scientific language.

For example, from the vertical curve lines in Figure 6 we can see that in the waveform of a periodicity of Gun Fa (rolling), an apparent epicycloidal wave is closely followed by an inward one whose mechanical quantity is as large as two-thirds of the former. This

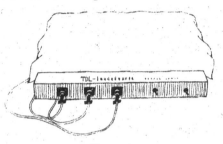

Figure 1

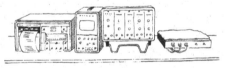

Figure 2

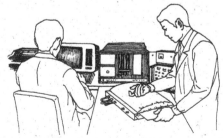

Figure 3

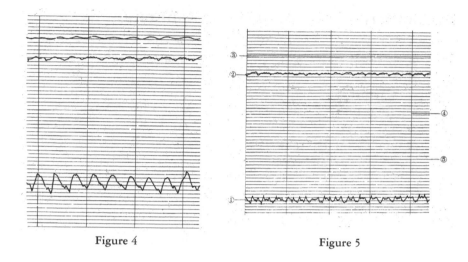

Figure 4

Figure 5

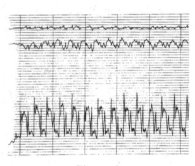

Figure 6

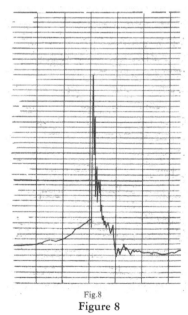

Fig.8
Figure 8

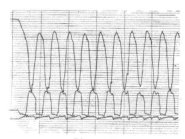

Figure 7

shows that the force exerted in one periodicity of Gun Fa is both outward and inward, giving the body two times stronger stimuli with one larger than the other. Therefore, compared with other manipulations, Gun Fa has larger stimulation quantity and rich mechanical information. This may be the reason that Gun Fa has certain advantages in treating diseases such as arthralgia, flaccidity, paralysis, and numbness.

Take Ping Tui Fa (translation-push), the main maneuver of Nei Gong Tuina, as another example. This maneuver seems just to push and rub the hand up and down over the operated part of the body, and beginners tend to direct their force horizontally. Yet is found out from the tri-dimensional dynamic-force curve lines supplied in Figure 7 that the proportions of the vertical, longitudinal, and transverse forces of Ping Tui Fa are 1:0.3:0. This makes it clear that the technical secret of Ping Tui Fa is to exert the force of the hand vertically on the operated part so as to lead its effect to the interior.

Obviously, this research has wide and practical value and academic significance. The research helps to:

- Sort the experience of the manipulations of modern physicians
- Develop tuina therapy
- Reform the traditional teaching methods (as needed)
- Study in greater depth the principles and mechanisms of the maneuvers of tuina manipulations

1.5 Schools of Tuina

Because of the long history and staged development of tuina, tuina has rich and colorful academic schools and systems that vary, for example, by specialty, region, and/or lineage of the teachers. A general study of the many schools discloses the fact that they are all the same in the following three ways:

1. Each has a long history and formed, spread, and thrived within a district
2. Each is guided by a theory, rich in medical practical experience, and has expert indications and unique methods for exercise and specialty training
3. Each has a main maneuver, which may be called "school maneuver," usually colored by evident touch of provincialism and local citizens.

Take Yi Zhi Chan Tuina (a manipulation operating with one thumb), for example.

- Yi Zhi Chan Tuina is popular in South China, especially in the provinces of Jiangsu and Zhejiang and the city of Shanghai, ever since the years of Xianfeng (an emperor) in the Qing Dynasty (1851-1862).

- It is operated according to the diagnosis made through comprehensively differentiating the all-round condition of both the syndrome and patient from the disease causing the distress.

- As for the maneuvers, the leading one is *yi zhi chan tui fa* (a manipulation operated with one thumb). The secondary maneuvers are *na* (grasping), *an* (pressing), *mo* (rubbing), *gun* (rolling), *nian* (twisting), *chao* (sweeping), *cuo* (foulage), *chan* (quick-push), *rou* (kneading), *yao* (rotating) and *dou* (shaking).

Yi Zhi Chan Tuina has a whole set of methods for training professional techniques. This school of tuina attaches special importance to learning basic skills because the leading maneuver and some secondary ones are hard to master.

This kind of tuina is mainly conducted along the fourteen channels, on the points along them, and on the extra-channel points and non-fixed points. It can be used to treat diseases, such as disorders of the channels, collaterals, body, or internal organs whether they are due to external or internal cause.

CHAPTER 2

Basics of Tuina

In ancient times, tuina did not distinguish between adult and infant patients. Since the Ming Dynasty (1368-1644), however, tuina developed to suit the physiological and pathological characteristics of infants. Later, adult tuina was advanced to distinguish it from infant tuina. Adult tuina is different from infant tuina in manipulation, stimulation quantity, selected points, therapeutic method, and indications. This book describes adult tuina in clinical practice. *Do NOT perform any of these manipulations on infants. Infant tuina is a therapy that requires advanced Eastern medical training and certification.*

2.1 Manipulations

While performing tuina, the practitioner concentrates his/her own mind, regulates the breath evenly, and moves the qi and power from all of his/her body to the hands. S/he keeps the power-bearing point on the operated part and manipulates the channels and points of the skin with certain standardized movements. Thus, tuina creates stimulating messages via a specific power pattern consisting of quantity, frequency, periodicity, rhythm, and direction of the manipulation's force. Each power pattern activates a specific function of the channels and their corresponding points. Like the ripple effect of a pebble thrown in the water, the effect of tuina manipulations "ripple" to different layers of body tissues from the points to superficial channels and collaterals to internal organs. In this way, the whole system enters an activated state in which optimal self-regulating functions are achieved. Therefore, tuina takes a therapeutic role in:
- Balancing yin and yang
- Restoring qi
- Removing excesses,
- Regulating ying and wei
- Smoothing the channels and collaterals
- Promoting the circulation of qi and blood

- Coordinating the zang and fu organs
- Relieving inflammation, stopping pain, lubricating the joints, etc.

In addition, tuina manipulations correct anatomic abnormalities and restore the function of injured soft tissues and tendons. For instance, when certain disorders—like displacement of muscle and tendon and/or subluxation of joints—are treated, different corresponding tuina maneuvers strengthen the body by regulating the *qi* flow and blood or treat the injured muscles and tendons by activating the channels and collaterals.

2.2 Characteristics of Manipulations and Point Selection of Tuina

Characteristics. The manipulations for tuina of any school are characterized by body region, motion range, and stimulation quantity. These characteristics are more suitable for application on an adult's body, including the points, the routes of the fourteen channels, and certain parts of the trunk or extremities.

Point Selection. The points selected for manipulation are usually on the superficial routes of the fourteen regular channels of the trunk and extremities, the extra-channel points, and the non-fixed points. The practitioner chooses the points and manipulations by differentiating the patient's age, sex, constitution, disease condition, and manipulated part. S/he puts the selected points and manipulations into order according to prescribed practice and then carries out the practical treatment. As for the rules and methods for selecting points, they are the same as those used in acupuncture therapy: local points, nearby points, distant points along the channel.

2.3 Commonly Used Mediums for Tuina

Mediums should be added when many tuina manipulations—Ca Fa (rub), Mo Fa (palm-rub), Ping Tui Fa (translation-push), and Zhi Tui Fa (finger-push)—are conducted in clinical practice. The effects of a medium is twofold:

1. To reinforce the effect of manipulations and raise curative effects through the action of the drugs it contains
2. To lubricate the manipulated skin of a patient, which benefits the performance of manipulations and protects the skin from being injured.

Nowadays, commonly used mediums for tuina include both traditional and contemporary mediums. A brief description of the more commonly used mediums follows:

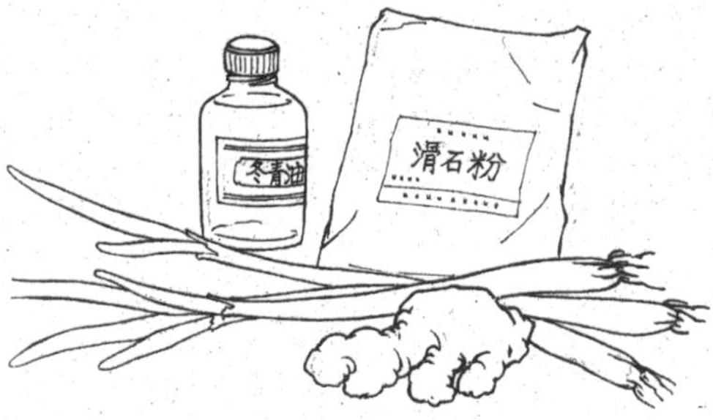

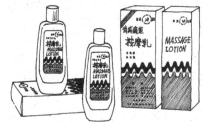

Figure 9

- Talcum Powder. Lubricates. Usually used in summer. When manipulations are conducted on parts where a lot of sweat tends to appear, local application of talcum powder may protect the skin of both the patient and the doctor (See Figure 9).

- Sesame Oil. Used in small quantity with Ca Fa (rubbing) to lubricate. Increases diathermic effect of the manipulation.

- Ointment of Chinese Holly Leaf. Made by mixing *dongqing* oil (methyl salicylate) with Vaseline. Used with Ca Fa (rub) or RouAnFa (knead-press). Strengthens the diathermic effect of the manipulations. Also removes wind-dampness, promotes blood circulation, and relieves pain (See Figure 9).

- Turpentine oil. Made from *honghua* (*Flos carthami*) and liquid medicine for relieving the rigidity of muscles. Activates collaterals.

- Massage Emulsion. Landing Stage (brand) Massage Emulsion manufactured by Jinan Chemical Plant for Producing Goods of Daily Use. Modern medium with natural perfume oil, extracts of herbal medicines, and surface-active agents. Clinical and pharmaco-logical experiments prove use with Mo (palm-rub) and Ca (rub), lubricates the skin and promotes blood circulation to stop pain, relieve inflammation, and alleviate fatigue (See Figure 10).

Figure 10

2.4 Points for Clinical Attention in Tuina

In tuina clinical practice, three factors are essential to ensure safe and effect treatment without side effects, facilitate practitioner's performance, and provide the patient with better medical service and mental ease. These factors include using essential medical facilities, preparation by and conduct of the practitioner and preparation by and conduct of the patient. Following is an explanation of each of the three factors.

Essential Medical Facilities:

- A spacious and bright consulting room in which there is fresh air, favorable temperature (25°C or so) and a convenient water supply.

- Beds that are clean, tidy, smooth, stable, fixed, not too high and not too low—reaching the knees of the practitioner is proper. Enough space around the bed so that the practitioner can regulate his/her standing position freely and do the work with ease.

- Accessibility to mediums—keep them ready within reach.

- Accessibility to appropriate medical towels, blankets, and soft cushions, which vary in size and are put beneath or on a patient's body during the course of treatment.

- Chairs or stools whose height may be easily adjusted.

- Large mirror(s) with lower edges are near the floor, in which the patient may look at him/herself when performing medical exercises.

Preparation by and Conduct of the Practitioner:

- Communication. Before treatment, a practitioner tells the patient with warm and sincere attitude about the treatment. This communication includes details about what responses are likely to happen while the manipulations are conducted and how s/he must cooperate. During the treatment, the practitioner interprets patiently what has happened in order to be trusted by the patient.

- Personal care. A practitioner often trims his/her fingernails, keeps his/her hands soft and smooth, and removes rings, watches and other jewelry from the hands before treatment lest the skin of the patient be injured.

- Observation. While s/he manipulates, the practitioner concentrates and observes attentively the patient's facial expressions and responses. S/he also pays close attention to the feeling of the hands. If and when something abnormal is found, timely proper measure is taken.

- Posture. According to the disease, constitution, age, sex, and manipulated part of the patient, the practitioner chooses an appropriate posture to ensure that the patient feels comfortable and that the manipulations are easily performed.

- Carrying out the Manipulations.

a. A practitioner pays attention to coordinating his/her own movements and brings his/her will, breathing, and maneuvers into line. Even when sudden exertion of strength is needed, do not hold or control your breathing to prepare for the exertion lest self-injuries occur.

b. Be sure the manipulated part is appropriately exposed. For example, Ping Tui Fa (translation-push) and Ca (rub) are performed directly on the patient's skin. Conversely, manipulations are performed through the patient's clothing or a towel in Yi Zhi Chan TuiFa (one-thumb operation) and GunFa (roll). If done otherwise, the manipulations' curative effects are lowered.

c. In the course of manipulation, the stimulation quantity and the passive motor scope is adjusted. It needs to be no smaller than necessary to reach the appropriate stimulation value, but as large as possible up to a point the patient can endure and the human structure, the pathological conditions, and the physiological function can stand.

Note: Violent manipulating will bring manipulative injuries to patients. As examples:

- Over-rubbing, over-pressing, digital-pressing, and over-kneading will break the skin and cause ecchymosis
- Violent hitting, beating, tapping, and pressing will lead to fracture and injury of the internal organs
- Over-pulling, over-rotating, and too much traction will result in laceration of ligaments and subluxation of joints
- Over-manipulating the spinal column will bring about subluxation of cervical vertebra, intimal laceration of the vertebral artery, and infarction of the cerebellum and brain stem

Preparation by and Conduct of the Patient:

- Trust. The patient trusts the practitioner, follows his/her orders, and cooperates with him/her closely.
- Exercise and diet. Patients do not go for the treatment after strenuous exercise or on a full or empty stomach. Optimally, treatment is given one hour after a meal and after at least ten minutes of rest in the consulting room.
- Near-time preparation. Just before treatment, the patient empties his/her bladder and removes outerwear and belt.
- Communication. The patient tells the practitioner about his/her health condition. S/he should include information

about fever, whether the skin is ruptured, damaged or infected near the part to be manipulated, and, she is menstruating or pregnant.

- State of mind. The patient calms the mind and relaxes the whole body. S/he should not read or go to sleep. S/he should pay attention to the experience of manipulation stimulation and tell the practitioner his/her feelings as the work is being done.

2.5 Indications of Tuina

2.5.1 DISORDERS DUE TO TRAUMA.

Indications of disorders due to trauma include:
- Various sprains and contusion
- Subluxation of joints
- Stiff neck
- Cervical spondylopathy
- Prolapse of lumbar intervertebral discs, posterior articular disturbance of lumbar vertebrae, or syndrome of the transverse process of the third lumbar vertebra
- Retrograde spondylitis
- Superior clunial neuritis
- Piriformis syndrome
- Scapulohumeral periarthritis
- Subacromial bursitis
- External humeral epicondylitis
- Tenosynovitis stenosans
- Meniscus injury
- Systremma
- Sternocostal shield injury
- Disturbance of costovertebral joints and functional disturbance of temporognathic joints

2.5.2 MEDICAL SYNDROMES.

Indications of disorders due to medical syndromes include:
- Epigastralgia
- Gastroptosis, gastrointestinal dysfunction, and gastroduodenal ulcer
- Headache

- Insomnia
- Asthma and pulmonary emphysema
- Cholecystitis
- Hypertension, angina pectoris, and coronary heart disease
- Diarrhea and constipation
- Diabetes
- Impotence
- Uroschesis
- Neurosism

2.5.3 DISEASE OF SURGERY.

Indications of surgical disorders include:
- Acute mastitis in the early stages
- Bed sore
- Post-operative intestinal adhesion

2.5.4 DISEASE OF GYNECOLOGY.

Indications of gynecological disorders include:
- Dysmenorrhea and irregular menstruation
- Anemia
- Pelvic inflammation
- Puerperal separation of symphysis pubis

2.6 Contraindications of Tuina

Contraindications of tuina include:
- Acute and chronic communicable diseases such as hepatitis
- Infective disease such as erysipelas, medullitis, and suppurative arthritis
- Various hemorrhagic diseases such as gastric ulcer in its bleeding period, hematochezia, and hematuria
- Various malignant tumors, tuberculosis, and pyemia
- Scald and localized area of ulcerative dermatitis
- Bleeding due to trauma
- Lumbosacral and abdominal portions of a woman in menstrual or pregnant period

CHAPTER 3

The Fourteen Channels and the Common Acupoints

According to Western medical principles, the explanation of why tuina is effective when treating diseases has not yet been clarified. We continue to explore mysteries such as the essence of channels and collaterals; the biomechanical feature of the movement of each tuina manipulation; and the bio-physiochemical process during which the stimulus of a manipulation is received, distributed, transformed, and utilized in the body. From TCM's point of view, the principles behind tuina's effectiveness focus on the effect produced when a manipulation is performed on the channel and point system of the human body. Based on energy flow and the relation of each part to the whole (of the body), TCM dictates that tuina's effectiveness depends on two simple sources: manipulations and channels.

All tuina clinical work such as differentiation and diagnosis of diseases, selection of points, composition of prescriptions, choice of manipulations, and operations of maneuvers are guided by the theory of channels and collaterals. *Therefore, the first thing for a student to do—even before practicing—is learn, understand, and remember the basic principles of the Fourteen Channels and the commonly used points.*

3.1 The Fourteen Channels

Literally, channel means "route," and collateral, "network." The channel is the cardinal conduit of the meridian system and the collateral is its branch. "Meridian" is the general term for both the channels and collaterals. The meridian system acts as specific passageways for the circulation of *qi* and blood throughout the body, the interconnection between visceral organs and extremities, and the communication of the upper body with the lower and of the interior body parts with the exterior. The channels take a definite route, but the collaterals are widely distributed throughout the body like an interlacing network that combines all structures of the body such as the *zang-fu* organs, body orifices, skin, muscles, tendons, and bones into an integral whole.

Channels and collaterals are everywhere in the whole body—in the organs and extremities. They connect all organs and tissues throughout the body such as *zang* (solid) organs, *fu* (hollow) organs, orifices, skin, tendons, muscles, and skeleton. *Qi* and blood circulate in the channels and collaterals, supply nutrients, and transmit messages from the interior to the exterior and vice versa. In this way, a whole stereoscopic regulating and controlling system is formed.

The term "Fourteen Channels" refers to the Twelve Regular Channels (those related to the 12 *zang-fu* organs), the Ren Channel, and the Du Channel.

3.1.1 THE TWELVE REGULAR CHANNELS.

The 12 channels are the main component of the system of the channels and collaterals. For this reason, they are also called "regular channels." Each corresponds to its respective *zang-fu* organ and is named after its respective *zang* or *fu* organ. For example, the channel connecting the heart is called Heart Channel; the one connecting the large intestine is the Large Intestine Channel, and so on.

In addition, all the channels belonging to *zang* are called *yin* channels, while those belonging to *fu* are *yang* channels.

Finally, there are also Three Yin Channels of Hand, Three Yin Channels of Foot, Three Yang Channels of Hand, and Three Yang Channels of Foot; these terms are given according to the distribution of the *yin* and *yang* channels in the upper and legs.

The Twelve Regular Channels are distributed on the body surface as follows.

- *Yang* channels are mainly distributed on the lateral surfaces of the arms and legs and on the back
- *Yin* channels are distributed on the medial surfaces of the arms and legs and on the abdominal portion (except that the Stomach Channel of Foot-Yangming crosses the trunk through the ventral surface)
- The Three Yin Channels of Hand start from the chest and run to the hand
- The Three Yang Channels of Hand run from the hand to the head

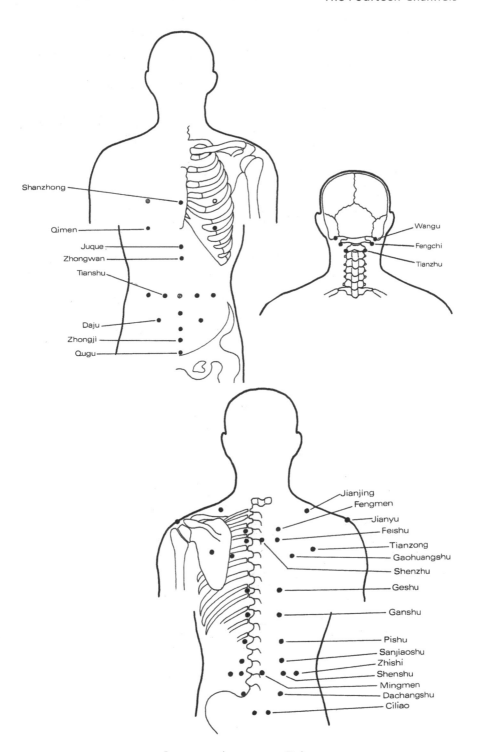

Important Acupressure Points

- The Three Yang Channels of Foot run from the head to the foot
- The Three Yin Channels of Foot run from the foot up to the abdomen
- The Twelve Regular Channels are connected to each other by their branches (collaterals).
- There are six pairs of connections among *zang* and *fu* organs and, correspondingly, six pairs of connections from the interior to the exterior among the *yin* and *yang* channels.
- *Yin* channels pertaining to *zang* but connected with *fu* and *yang* channels pertaining to *fu* but connected to *zang* are linked together through the Channels of Hand and Foot. This system starts from the Lung Channel, ends at the Liver Channel and starts again from the Lung Channel, just like a ring in which *qi* and blood circulate endlessly.

See the diagram below for a visual representation of the relationships and paths of the channels and collaterals.

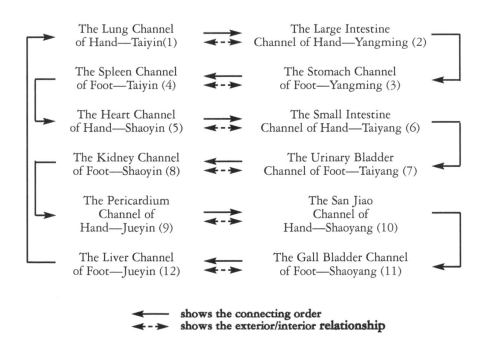

The Lung Channel of Hand—Taiyin(1)	The Large Intestine Channel of Hand—Yangming (2)
The Spleen Channel of Foot—Taiyin (4)	The Stomach Channel of Foot—Yangming (3)
The Heart Channel of Hand—Shaoyin (5)	The Small Intestine Channel of Hand—Taiyang (6)
The Kidney Channel of Foot—Shaoyin (8)	The Urinary Bladder Channel of Foot—Taiyang (7)
The Pericardium Channel of Hand—Jueyin (9)	The San Jiao Channel of Hand—Shaoyang (10)
The Liver Channel of Foot—Jueyin (12)	The Gall Bladder Channel of Foot—Shaoyang (11)

◀——— shows the connecting order
◀-► shows the exterior/interior **relationship**

Physiologically, the Twelve Regular Channels function in primarily three ways:

1. To connect all parts of the body. Channels are the direct passages in the system of the channels and collaterals, while collaterals are a network of branches of every kind connecting the channels and organs. These organs include the five *zang*, six *fu*, limbs, bones, skin, muscles, tendons, and the five sense organs.

2. To transport *qi* and blood. The channels and collaterals crisscross throughout the body, forming a system in which *qi* and blood circulate and bring nutrients to the tissues and organs of all parts of the body so as to maintain the normal physiological function of the human body.

3. To regulate the function of the body. Because of both the crisscross connections and the regulation function of the channels and collaterals, all parts of the body can work cooperatively so that the invasion of pathogenic factors are resisted and the body functions normally. In fact, if the organism is in a state of pathology, the channels and collaterals signal the symptoms and signs and transmit the route of diseases. Diseases attacking the internal organs may be manifested on the body's surface through the channels and collaterals. For example, tenderness, allergic reaction, or other pathological manifestations may occur on a specific part of the body surface after some visceral diseases develop. Injuries and disorders of the body surface may also affect the internal tissues and organs at any level through the system of the channels and collaterals. Disease of one organ may lead to disease of another organ, again because of their connections of channels and collaterals.

3.1.2 THE REN CHANNEL AND THE DU CHANNEL

The channels of Ren, Du, Chong, Dai, Yangqiao, Yinqiao, Yangwei and Yinwei collectively are called the Eight Extraordinary (or Extra) Channels. They are different from the Twelve Regular Channels in that they neither pertain to *zang-fu* organs directly nor have exterior-interior relationship with any other channel. Their main physiological function is to regulate *qi* and blood in the Twelve Regular Channels.

1. The Ren Channel runs along the midline of the abdomen and chest and up to the mandible. On the way, it meets the *yin* channels of the whole body. That is why it is called the "sea of *yin* channels." It regulates *qi* in all the *yin* channels.

2. The Du Channel runs along the midline of the waist, back, and nape and up to the cranium. On the way, it meets the *yang* channels of the whole body. That is why it is called "the sea of *yang* channels." It regulates *qi* in all the *yang* channels. Of the Eight Extra Channels, only the Ren and Du Channels have their own points. All the other six share points of the 12 Regular Channels. Because they have their own points, the Ren and Du Channels are included with the 12 Regular Channels to form the Fourteen Channels as the basis of tuina therapy.

3.2 The Acupoints

Locations where *qi* and blood of the channels, collaterals, and viscera come in, go out, and pool by way of transfusion are called points. They fall into the following three categories:

1. Channel points have specific names and locations on the route of any of the fourteen channels

2. Extraordinary points have specific names and locations **not** on the route of any of the fourteen channels

3. *Ashi* points or *tianying* points do not have specific names or locations. They are located according to where there is tenderness or other reactions.

All the points, no matter what kind they are, are closely related to the channels and collaterals, and by means of the channels and collaterals, they closely connect with the *zang* and *fu* organs and the tissues of the whole body. They reflect the physiological and pathological changes of the organs and tissues so as to provide a basis for clinical differentiation, diagnosis, selection of tuina points, and composition of tuina prescription.

The points also serve as the stimulated spots of tuina manipulations. Stimulating the points with manipulation is intended to stimulate the adjusting function of the corresponding channels and collaterals so that the function of *qi* and blood of the *zang-fu* organs can be regulated. This helps the inherent ability of the body to resist diseases.

Identifying the correct tuina points directly affects the curative effects in clinical practice. To ensure right locations of the points, sound methods are needed. Following are commonly used methods of identification.

3.2.1 PROPORTIONAL MEASUREMENTS.

The width or length of various portions of the human body is divided respectively into definite numbers of equal units. Each unit is divided respectively into definite numbers of equal subunits, each of which is called one *cun*. The method to locate points with this measurement is called proportional measurements. This method is applicable to patients of different ages and body sizes. (See Figure 11 and the following table to find into how many *cun* each portion of the body is divided.).

3.2.2 FINGER MEASUREMENT

This is a method used to locate points with the length or width of the patient's finger(s). The practitioner's finger(s) may be used instead if

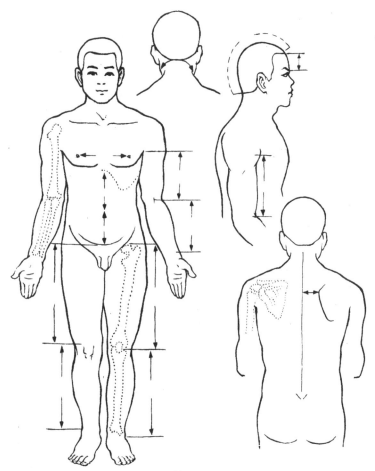

Figure 11

Body Part	Distance	Proportional Measurement	Method	Explanation
Head	From the anterior hairline to the posterior hairline.	12 *Cun*	Longitudinal Measurement	The Distance from the glabella to the anterior hairline is taken as 3 *Cun*; from the Dazhui (DU14) to the posterior hairline, 3 *Cun*. If the anterior and posterior hairlines are indistinguishable, the distance from the glabella to the Dazhui (DU14) is then taken as 18 *Cun*.
Chest and Abdomen	Between the two nipples.	8 *Cun*	Transverse Measurement	The distance between the bilateral Quepen (ST12) can be used as the substitute of the transverse measurement of the two nipples.
	From the end of the Xiphoid process to the center of the umbilicus.	8 *Cun*	Longitudinal Measurement	
	Between the center of the umbilicus and the upper margin of pubic bone.	5 *Cun*	Longitudinal Measurement	
Back	Between the medial borders of the two scapulae.	6 *Cun*	Transverse Measurement	Transverse measurement used to locate points on the loins and back.

Upper Extremities	Between the end of the axillary fold and the transverse cubital crease.	9 *Cun*	Longitudinal Measurement	Applicable to the measurement of both the medial and lateral aspects of the upper limb.
	Between the transverse cubital crease and transverse wrist crease.	12 *Cun*	Longitudinal Measurement	
Lower Extremities	From the prominence of the great trochanter to the middle of the patella.	19 *Cun*	Longitudinal Measurement	For measurement of the thigh.	For measurement of the anterior, lateral and posterior aspects of the lower limbs.
	Between the center of the patella and the tip of the lateral malleolus.	16 *Cun*	Longitudinal Measurement	For measurement of the shank.
	From the level of the upper margin of pubic bone to the upper border of the medial epicondylic ridge.	18 *Cun*	Longitudinal Measurement	For measurement of the thigh.	For measurement of the medial aspects of the lower limbs.
	From the lower border of the medial condyle of the tibia to the tip of the medial malleolus.	13 *Cun*	Longitudinal Measurement	For measurement of the shank.

Table 1

his/her body size is similar to that of the patient. Generally speaking, when the patient's middle finger is flexed, the distance between both medial ends of the creases of the interphalangeal joints is taken as one *cun* or the width of the interphalangeal joint of the patient's thumb is taken as one *cun*. In addition, the width of the proximal interphalangeal joints of the closed four fingers (index, middle, ring, and small) is taken as three *cun* (See Figure 12-1 and 12-2).

3.3.3 Measurement Based on Anatomical Landmarks

Locating points according to various anatomical landmarks on the body surface is a basic method for point location. Those landmarks fall into two categories: fixed and moving.

Fixed Landmarks. Fixed landmarks are those whose positions will not change with body movement. The five sense organs, nipples, umbilicus, and the protrusions and depressions of various bones are examples of fixed landmarks.

Moving Landmarks. Moving Landmarks refer to those that will appear only when a body part remains in a specific position. The depression and prominence of the muscles, the appearance of the tendons, and the creases of the skin when a movement is being done are examples.

3.3 The Channels and Points Commonly Used in Tuina Manipulations

3.3.1 The Lung Channel of Hand-Taiyin

This channel originates from the middle-*jiao*, runs downward to

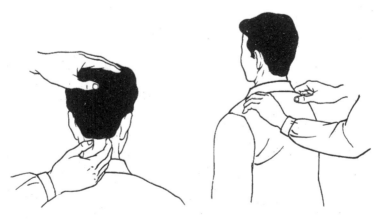

Figure 12-1 Figure 12-2

connect with the large intestine, winds back and goes upward into the lung—the organ to which it pertains—comes out transversely from the lung system to reach Zhongfu (LU 1), descends along the radial border of the medial aspect of the arm, and ends at Shaoshang (LU 11) at the radial side of the thumb. Its branch emerging from Lieque (LU 7) runs to the radial side of the tip of the index finger, where it meets the Large Intestine Channel of Hand-Yangming, to which the Lung Channel of Hand-Taiyin is exteriorly-interiorly related. Located along either of the left or right routes of the Lung Channel of Hand-Taiyin are 11 points. Following are the most commonly used of these 11 points. (See Figure 13).

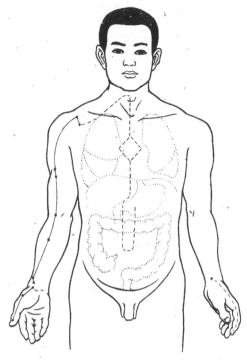

Figure 13

1. Zhongfu (LU 1)

   a. Location: 6 *cun* lateral to the midline of the chest, at the level of the interspace between the 1st and 2nd ribs

   b. Indications: Cough, choking sensation in the chest, chest pain, and pain in the shoulder and back

   c. Manipulations: Yizhichan Tui, An, Rou, and Mo

2. Chize (LU 5)

   a. Location: In the middle of the cubital crease and on the radial side of the tendon of the biceps muscle of the arm.

   b. Indications: Spasmodic pain of the elbow and arm, cough, fullness in the chest and the hypochondriac region, and infantile convulsions

   c. Manipulations: An, Rou, Na and Yizhichan Tui

3. Lieque (LU 7)

   a. Location: Superior to the styloid process of the radius, 1.5 *cun* above the transverse crease of the wrist. When the index fingers and thumbs of both hands are crossed with the index finger of one hand placed on the styloid process of the radius of the other, the point is in the depression right under the tip of the index finger.

b. Indications: Headache, facial paralysis and hemiplegia

c. Manipulations: An and Qia (nip).

4. Yuji (LU 10)

a. Location: At the midpoint of the first metacarpal bone and on the junction of the red and white skin

b. Indications: Pain in the chest and back, headache, vertigo, sore throat, and fever with chills

c. Manipulations: An, Rou, and Qia

5. Shashang (LU 11)

a. Location: On the radial side of the thumb and about 1 *cun* posterior to the corner of the nail

b. Indications: Swollen and sore throat, cough with dyspnea, apoplexy, coma, and infantile convulsions

c. Manipulations: Qia and Qiarou (nip-knead).

3.3.2 THE LARGE INTESTINE CHANNEL OF HAND-YANGMING

This channel originates from Shangyang (LI 1) on the radial side of the index finger, runs upward along the radial border of the lateral side of the hand and arm to the anterior border of the acromion, winds backward and reaches Dazhui (DU 14), turns back and arrives at the supraclavicular fossa, descends to the pass through the lung, and at last enters the large intestine—the organ to which it belongs. Its branch starts from the supraclavicular fossa, goes upward to the neck, passes through the cheek and the gum of the lower teeth, winds backward to the upper lip, meets Renzhong (DU 26), goes forward again, and ends at Yingxiang (LI 20), at which point it connects with the Stomach Channel of Foot-Yangming. The Large Intestine Channel of Hand-Yangming is exteriorly-interiorly related to the Lung Channel. Along the each the left and right route, there are 20 points. The commonly used ones are as follows (See Figure 14).

1. Hegu (LI 4)

a. Location: On the dorsum of the hand and at the midpoint between the 1st and 2nd metacarpal bones

b. Indications: Headache, toothache, fever, swollen and sore throat, pain in the shoulder and arm, finger spasm, and facial paralysis

   c. Manipulations: Na, An,
   and RouQia (knead-nip).
2. Yangxi (LI 5)

   a. Location: On the radial
   transverse crease of the
   dorsum of the wrist and
   between the vagina
   *tendinum musculorum
   abductoris longi et exten-
   soris brevis policis* and
   tendinous sheath of long
   extensor muscle of
   thumb

   b. Indications: Headache,
   tinnitus, toothache,
   swollen and sore throat,
   conjunctival congestion,
   and wrist pain

   c. Manipulations: An, Rou,
   Qia, and Na

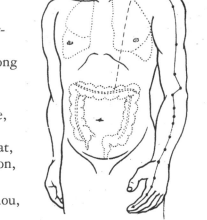

Figure 14

3. Shousanli (LI 10)

   a. Location: 2 *cun* below
   quchi (LI 11) and on the line between *yangxi* (LI 5) and *quchi*
   (LI 11)

   b. Indications: Spasmodic elbow with difficulty in flexion and
   extension, and numbness and soreness of the arm

   c. Manipulations: Na, An, Rou, and Yizhichan Tui

4. Quchi (LI 11)

   a. Location: In the depression at the lateral end of the cubital
   transverse crease when the elbow is flexed

   b. Indications: Fever, hypertension, swollen and painful elbow
   and arm with difficulty in flexion and extension, and paralysis

   c. Manipulations: Na, An, Rou, and Qia.

5. Jianyu (LI 15)

   a. Location: In the depression anterior and inferior to the
   acromion when the arm is abducted

   b. Indications: Pain in the shoulder, motor impairment of the
   shoulder, and hemiparalysis

   c. Manipulations: Yizhichan Tui, An, Rou and Gun

6. Yingxiang (LI 20)

    a. Location: In the nasolabial groove and at the point 0.5 *cun* lateral to the ala nas*i*.

    b. Indications: Rhinitis, stuffy nose, and facial paralysis

    c. Manipulations: Qia, An, Rou, and Yizhichan Tui

3.3.3. THE STOMACH CHANNEL OF FOOT-YANGMING

This channel originates from the lateral side of the ala nasi, runs upward to meet the Bladder Channel of Foot-Taiyang at the radix nasi and arrives at Chengqi (ST 1) at the infraorbital margin, descends through the upper gum, around the lips and along the mandible and Jiache (ST 6), and finally winds upward again to reach Touwei (ST 8) at the preauricular frontal angle. The facial branch starts from the mandible, descends into the supraclavicular fossa along the neck, descends again and passes through the diaphragm, enters the stomach—the organ to which it pertains—and connects with the spleen. The branch travelling along the exterior route starts from the supraclavicular fossa, descends through the nipple and abdomen, meets the branch arising from the lower orifice of the stomach at Qichong (ST 30), runs downward again along the anterior side of the thigh and the anterolateral aspect of the tibia, and ends at Lidui (ST 45) on the second toe. Located along this channel and on both its routes are 90 points. The following are commonly used. This channel is exteriorly-interiorly related to the Spleen Channel (See Figure 15).

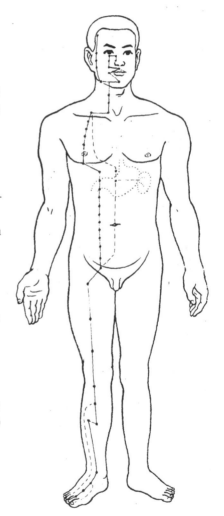

Figure 15

1. Sibai (ST 2)

   a. Location: In the depression of the infraorbital forearm and directly below the pupil while one is looking straight ahead

   b. Indication: Facial paralysis; spasm of the facial muscles; and reddened, painful and itchy eye(s)

   c. Manipulations: An, Rou, and Yizhichan Tui

2. Dicang (ST 4)

   a. Location: 0.4 *cun* lateral to the corner of the mouth, directly below Juliao (ST 3)

   b. Indications: Facial paralysis and salivation

   c. Manipulations: Yizhichan Tui, An, and Rou

3. Jiache (ST 6)

   a. Location: In the depression one finger-breadth anterior and superior to the lower angle of the mandible

   b. Indications: Toothache, swelling of the cheek, and facial paralysis

   c. Manipulations: Yizhichan Tui, An, and Rou

4. Xiaguan (ST 7)

   a. Location: In the depression on the lower border of the zygomatic arch

   b. Indications: Facial paralysis, toothache, and temporomandibular joint inflammation

   c. Manipulations: Yizhichan Tui, An, and Rou

5. Touwei (ST 8)

   a. Location: 0.5 *cun* directly above the anterior hairline at the corner of the forehead

   b. Indications: Headache, Vertigo and ophthalmalgia

   c. Manipulations: Mo, An, Rou, and Saosan (knead-sweep)

6. Renying (ST 9)

   a. Location: 1.5 *cun* lateral to the laryngeal protuberance

   b. Indications: Swollen and sore throat, asthma, choking sensation in the chest, emesis, and hiccups

   c. Manipulations: Na, Rou, and Chan (twining)

7. Shuitu (ST 10)

   a. Location: 1 *cun* inferior to Renying (ST 9) and on the anterior border of *m. sternocleidomastoideus*

   b. Indications: Fullness in the chest, cough, asthma, swollen and sore throat, and shortness of breath

   c. Manipulations: Na, Mo, and Chan

8. Quepen (ST 12)

   a. Location: In the depression of the midpoint of supraclavicular fossa and directly above the nipple

   b. Indications: Fullness in the chest, cough, asthma, sore throat, and pain and numbness in the arm.

   c. Manipulations: An, Tanbo (flick-poke) and Rou.

9. Tianshu (ST 25)

   a. Location: 2 *cun* lateral to the umbilicus

   b. Indications: Constipation, diarrhea, irregular menstruation, and abdominal pain

   c. Manipulations: Rou, Mo, and Yizhichan Tui

10. Biguan (ST 31)

   a. Location: On the line jointing the anterior superior iliac spine and the lateral border of the patella and at the level of the gluteal groove

   b. Indications: Soreness of the loins and legs, numbness and weakness of the legs with spasmodic tendons that lead to difficulty in flexion and extension, and myoatrophy of the quadriceps muscle of thigh

   c. Manipulations: An, Na, Rou, DiAn, Gun and Tanbo

11. Futu (ST 32)

   a. Location: 6 *cun* above the laterosuperior border of the patella

   b. Indications: Pain, coldness and numbness of the knee, and paralysis of the legs

   c. Manipulations: Gun, An, and Rou

12. Liangqiu (ST 34)

   a. Location: 2 *cun* above the laterosuperior border of the patella

   b. Indications: Pain, coldness and numbness of the knee, stomachache, and mastitis.

   c. Manipulations: Gun, An, DiAn, and Na

13. Dubi (ST 35)

   a. Location: In the depression lateral to the patellar ligament and on the lower border of the patella

   b. Indications: Pain, weakness, and motor impairment of the knee

   c. Manipulations: DiAn, An, and Rou

14. Zusanli (ST 36)

    a. Location: 3 *cun* below Dubi (ST 35), one finger-breadth apart from the anterior crest of the tibia

    b. Indications: Abdominal pain and distension, diarrhea, constipation, coldness and numbness in the legs, and hypertension

    c. Manipulations: An, DiAn, Rou, and Yizhichan Tui

15. Shangjuxu (ST 37)

    a. Location: 3 *cun* directly below Zusanli (ST 36)

    b. Indications: Pain around the navel, diarrhea, appendicitis, soreness and numbness in the legs, and paralysis

    c. Manipulations: An, Na, Gun, and Rou

16. Jiexi (ST 41)

    a. Location: On the dorsum of the foot, at the midpoint of the transverse crease of the ankle, in the depression between the tendon of *m. extensor digorum longus* and *hallucis longus*

    b. Indications: Ankle sprain, numbness of the foot and toes, and headache

    c. Manipulations: An, Na, Qia, and DiAn

3.3.4. THE SPLEEN CHANNEL OF FOOT-TAIYIN

This channel originates from Yinbai (SP 1) at the tip of the big toe, runs along the medial aspect of the foot, goes upward from the medial aspect of the ankle, ascends along the anterior border of the medial aspects of the tibia and the thigh up to Chongmen (SP 12) in the groin. The exterior route runs upward into the abdomen, ascends along a line 2 *cun* lateral to the midline of the abdomen to the chest, and then descends to Dabao (SP 21) at the hypochondrium. The interior route runs inside, enters the spleen—the organ to which it pertains—and connects with the stomach, then ascends alongside the esophagus, and finally reaches the root of the tongue and spreads over the lower surface of the tongue. The branch arising from the stomach goes upwards, passes through the diaphragm, enters the heart, and connects with the Heart Channel of Hand-Shaoyin. This channel is exteriorly-interiorly related to the Stomach Channel. Located along either of the left and right routes are 21 points, of which the following are commonly used (See Figure 16).

    1. Gongsun (SP 4)

        a. Location: On the medial aspect of the tarsal bones of the foot, in the depression of the anterior and inferior border of the base of the first metatarsal bone

b. Indications: Diarrhea, abdominal pain, vomiting, and swelling and pain on the medial aspect of the foot

c. Manipulations: An, Rou, DiAn, and Yizhichan Tui

2. Sanyinjiao (SP 6)

a. Location: 3 *cun* directly above the tip of the medial malleolus, on the posterior border of the medial aspect of the tibia

b. Indications: Insomnia, enuresis, weakness of the spleen and stomach, uroschesis, nocturnal emission, impotence, irregular menstruation, and hypertension

c. Manipulations: Rou, An, and Yizhichan Tui

3. Yinlingquan (SP 9)

a. Location: In the depression of the hypocondylar border on the medial aspect of the tibia

b. Indications: Soreness of the knee and difficulty in urinating

c. Manipulations: Rou, An, DiAn, Na, and Yizhichan Tui

4. Xuehai (SP 10)

a. Location: 2 *cun* above the mediosuperior border of the patella

b. Indications: Irregular menstruation and soreness of the knee

c. Manipulations: Na, An, and DiAn

5. Daheng (SP 15)

a. Location: 4 *cun* lateral to the center of the umbilicus

b. Indications: Diarrhea due to cold of insufficiency type constipation and pain in the lower abdomen

c. Manipulations: Yizhichan Tui, Mo, Rou, and Na

3.3.5. THE HEART CHANNEL OF HAND-SHAOYIN

This channel originates from the heart, spreads over the heart system—

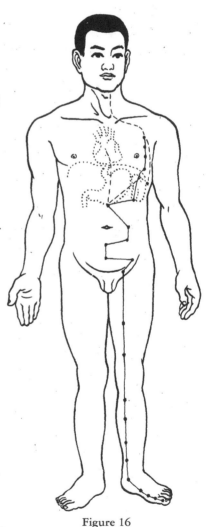

Figure 16

the tissues connecting the heart with the other *zang-fu* organs—and descends to connect with the small intestine. The portion of this channel ascending from the heart system runs alongside the esophagus to connect the eye and the tissues that connect the eye with the brain. The other portion of this channel coming out of the heart system runs upward to the lung, goes transversely to the left and right, emerges from Jiquan (HT 1) at the axilla, travels downward along the upper arm, the elbow and the palmar ulnar border of the forearm into the palm, ends at Shaochong (HT 9) at the tip of the medial aspect of the small finger and links with the Small Intestine Channel of Hand-Taiyang. This channel is exteriorly-interiorly related to the Small Intestine Channel. Along it, there are 18 points, nine on the left route, nine on the right route. The following are its commonly used points (See Figure 17).

1. Jiquan (HT 1)

   a. Location: In the center of the axilla

   b. Indications: Choking sensation in the chest; pain in the hypochondriac region; and soreness, coldness, and numbness of the arm and elbow

   c. Manipulations: Na and Tanbo

2. Shaohai (HT 3)

   a. Location: When the elbow is flexed, the point is located in the depression of the ulnar end of the transverse cubital crease

   b. Indications: Spasmodic pain in the elbow and tremor of the hand

   c. Manipulations: Na and Tanbo

3. Shenmen (HT 7)

   a. Location: At the ulnar end of the transverse crease of the wrist, in the depression on the

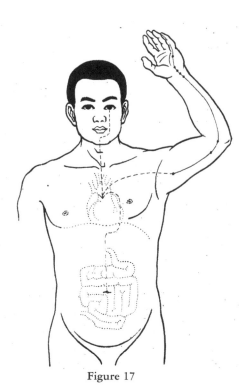

Figure 17

radial side of the tendon of *m. flexor carpi ulnaris*

b. Indications: Palpitation due to fright, severe palpitation, insomnia, amnesia, and arrhythmia

c. Manipulations: Na, An, and Rou

3.3.6. THE SMALL INTESTINE CHANNEL OF HAND-TAIYANG.

This channel originates from Shaoze (SI 1) on the ulnar side of the tip of the small finger, runs upward along the ulnar border of the dorsum of the hand and forearm to the shoulder, circles around the scapular region and goes further to meet Dazhui (DU 14), turns downward to Quepen (ST 12) in the supraclavicular fossa. From there, the inside branch descends to connect with the heart and further to enter the small intestine—the organ to which it belongs. The branch going superficially from the supraclavicular fossa ascends to the neck and further to the cheek, enters the ear, and ends

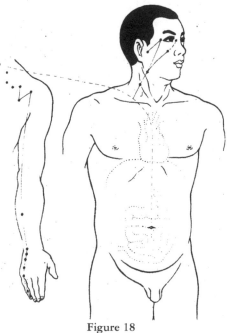

Figure 18

at Tinggong (SI 19). The branch from the neck runs upward to the infraorbital region and further to the lateral side of the nose, reaches the inner canthus and links with the Bladder Channel of Foot-Taiyang. The Small Intestine Channel of Hand-Taiyang is exteriorly-interiorly related to the Heart Channel. Located along it are 38 points, 19 on the left route and 19 on the right route. The commonly used ones are as follows (See Figure 18).

1. Shaoze (SI 1)

a. Location: On the ulnar side of the small finger, about 0.1 *cun* posterior to the corner of the nail

b. Indications: Fever, coma due to apoplexy, hypogalactia, and sore throat

c. Manipulations: Qia

2. Xiaohai (SI 8)

a. Location: In the depression between the olecranon of the ulna and the medial epicondyle of the humerus when the elbow is flexed

b. Indications: Toothache, pain in the neck and soreness in the arms

c. Manipulations: Na and Rou

3. Bingfeng (SI 12)

a. Location: In the center of the suprascapular fossa, directly above Tianzong (SI 11)

b. Indications: Pain in the scapular region and soreness and numbness in the arms with difficulty in raising them

c. Manipulations: Yizhichan Tui, Gun, An, and Rou

4. Jianwaishu (SI 14)

a. Location: 3 *cun* lateral to the lower border of the spinous process of the first thoracic vertebra

b. Indications: Cold pain in the shoulder and back, rigidity of the neck, and soreness and numbness in the arms

c. Manipulations: Yizhichan Tui, Gun, An, and Rou

5. Jianzhongshu (SI 15)

a. Location: 2 *cun* lateral to Dazhui (DU 14)

b. Indications: Cough, asthma, pain in the shoulder and back, and blurred vision

c. Manipulations: Yizhichan Tui, Gun, An, and Rou

6. Jianzhen (SI 9)

a. Location: 1 *cun* above the posterior end of the axillary fold

b. Indications: Soreness and motor impairment of the shoulder and arm paralysis

c. Manipulations: Gun, An, DiAn, Rou, and Na

7. Tianzong (SI 11)

a. Location: in between the infrafossa of the spine and scapula

b. Indications: Soreness of the shoulder and back; motor impairment of the shoulder; rigidity of the neck; and pain and numbness in the arm

c. Manipulations: Yizhichan Tui, Gun, An, DiAn, and Rou

8. Quanliao (SI 18)

a. Location: Directly below the outer canthus, in the depression on the lower border of the zygoma

b. Indications: Facial paralysis and facial spasm

c. Manipulations: Yizhichan Tui, Rou, An, and DiAn

3.3.7. THE BLADDER CHANNEL OF FOOT-TAIYANG.

This channel starts from Jingming (BL 1) at the inner canthus, ascends via the forehead and meets the Du Channel at the vertex (where a branch arises, running to the temple). From there, it goes inside to communicate with the brain, comes out and descends along the posterior aspect of the neck, runs downward alongside the medial aspect of the scapula and parallel to the vertebral column to the lumbar region (where another branch arises, descending). From there, it goes inside the body cavity, connects with the kidney and enters the urinary bladder—the organ to which it pertains.

The branch from the lumbar region descends via the buttock into the popliteal fossa.

There is yet another branch arising from the posterior aspect of the neck. It runs straight downward along the medial border of the scapula, passes the buttock and the lateral aspect of the thigh, meets the branch from the lumbar region in the popliteal fossa. From there, it makes its way downward via the shank, emerges from the posterior aspect of the lateral malleolus, runs along the tuberosity of the fifth metatarsal bone, and ends at Zhiyin (BL 67) at the lateral side of the tip of the small toe, where it connects with the Kidney Channel of Foot-Shaoyin.

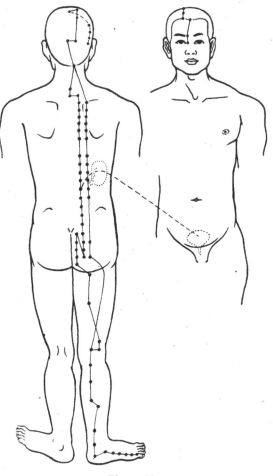

Figure 19

The Bladder Channel of Foot-Taiyang is exteriorly-interiorly related to the Kidney Channel. Along it, there are 134 points located all over the body, every two of which share the same name. The commonly used ones are as follows (See Figure 19).

1. Jimgming (BL 1)

   a. Location: 0.1 *cun* lateral to the inner canthus

   b. Indications: Eye disorders

   c. Manipulations: Yizhichan Tui, An, and Zhen

2. Cuanzhu (BL 2)

   a. Location: In the depression on the medial extremity of the eyebrow

   b. Indications: Headache, insomnia, supraorbital pain, and eye redness and pain

   c. Manipulations: Yizhichan Tui, An, Rou, and Mo

3. Tianzhu (BL 10)

   a. Location: 1.3 *cun* lateral to Yamen (DU 15), in the depression on the lateral border of *m. trapezius*

   b. Indications: Headache, rigidity of the neck, stuffy nose, and pain in the shoulder and back

   c. Manipulations: Yizhichan Tui, An, Rou, and Na

4. Dazhu (BL 11)

   a. Location: 1.5 *cun* lateral to the lower border of the spinous process of the first thoracic vertebra

   b. Indications: Fever, cough, neck rigidity, and pain in the shoulder and back

   c. Manipulations: Yizhichan Tui, Gun, An, and Rou

5. Fengmen (BL 12)

   a. Location: 1.5 *cun* lateral to the lower border of the spinous process of the second thoracic vertebra

   b. Indication: Cold, cough, neck rigidity, and pain in the shoulder and back

   c. Manipulations: Yizhichan Tui, Gun, An, and Rou

6. Feishu (BL 13)

   a. Location: 1.5 *cun* lateral to the lower border of the spinuous process of the third thoracic vertebra

   b. Indications: Cough, asthma, stuffiness and pain in the chest, and strained back muscles

   c. Manipulations: Yizhichan Tui, Gun, An, Rou, and Tanbo

7. Xinshu (BL 15)

    a. Location: 1.5 *cun* lateral to the lower border of the spinous process of the fifth thoracic vertebra

    b. Indications: Insomnia, amnesia, hemiparalysis, palpitation, and irritability

    c. Manipulations: Yizhichan Tui, Gun, An, Rou, and Tanbo.

8. Ganshu (BL 18)

    a. Location: 1.5 *cun* lateral to the lower border of the spinous process of the ninth thoracic vertebra

    b. Indications: Distending pain in the hypochondriac region, hepatitis, and eye disorders

    c. Manipulations: Yizhichan Tui Gun, An, Rou, and Tanbo

9. Danshu (BL 19)

    a. Location: 1.5 *cun* lateral to the lower border of the spinous process of the tenth thoracic vertebra

    b. Indications: Distending and full sensation in the hypochondriac region, bitter taste in the mouth, jaundice, and biliary tract disorders

    c. Manipulations: Yizhichan Tui, An, Rou, and Tanbo

10. Pishu (BL 20)

    a. Location: 1.5 *cun* lateral to the lower border of the spinous process of the eleventh thoracic vertebra

    b. Indications: Distending pain in the epigastric region, indigestion, and chronic infantile convulsion

    c. Manipulations: Yizhichan Tui, DiAn, An, and Rou

11. Weishu (BL 21)

    a. Location: 1.5 *cun* lateral to the lower border of the spinous process of the twelfth thoracic vertebra

    b. Indications: Gastropathy, vomiting of milk in infants, and indigestion

    c. Manipulations: Yizhichan Tui, DiAn, An, Rou, and Gun

12. Sanjiaoshu (BL 22)

    a. Location: 1.5 *cun* lateral to the lower border of the spinous process of the 1st lumbar vertebra

    b. Indications: Borborygmus, abdominal distension, vomiting, and rigidity and pain in the waist and back

    c. Manipulations: Yizhichan Tui, An, Rou, DiAn, and Gun

13. Shenshu (BL 23)

   a. Location: 1.5 *cun* lateral to the lower border of the spinous process of the 2nd lumbar vertebra

   b. Indications: Deficient kidney, lumbago, nocturnal emission, and irregular menstruation

   c. Manipulations: Yizhichan Tui, Gun, An, Rou, and DiAn

14. Qihaishu (BL 24)

   a. Location: 1.5 *cun* lateral to the lower order of the spinous process of the 3rd lumbar vertebra

   b. Indications: Lumbago and hemorrhoids

   c. Manipulations: Yizhichan Tui, An, Rou, and Gun

15. Dachangshu (BL 25)

   a. Location: 1.5 *cun* lateral to the lower border of the spinous process of the 4th lumbar vertebra

   b. Indications: Pain in the loins and legs, lumbar muscle strain, and enteritis

   c. Manipulations: Yizhichan Tui, An, Rou, and Gun

16. Guanyuanshu (BL 26)

   a. Location: 1.5 *cun* lateral to the lower border of the spinous process of the 5th lumbar vertebra

   b. Indications: Lumbago and diarrhea

   c. Manipulations: Yizhichan Tui, An, Gun, Rou, and DiAn

17. Zhibian (BL 54)

   a. Location: 3 *cun* lateral to the lower border of the spinous process of the 4th sacral vertebra

   b. Indications: Pain in the lumbosacral region, flaccidity of the lower extremities, difficulty in micturition, and constipation

   c. Manipulations: Gun, Na, An, Rou, DiAn, and Tanbo

18. Yinmen (BL 37)

   a. Location: 6 *cun* below the center of the gluteal groove

   b. Indications: Sciatica, paralysis of the lower extremities, and pain in the loins and legs

   c. Manipulations: Gun, DiAn, Ya (heavy pressing), and Na

19. Weizhong (BL 40)

   a. Location: At the midpoint of the transverse crease of the popliteal fossa

   b. Indications: Lumbago, difficulty in flexing and extending the knee, and hemiparalysis

      c. Manipulations: Gun, Na, An, Rou, and Yizhichan Tui

20. Gaohuang (BL 34)

      a. Location: 3 *cun* lateral to the lower border of the spinous process of the 4th thoracic vertebra, in the depression on the spinal border of the scapula

      b. Indications: Cough, asthma, tidal fever, mania, amnesia, and nocturnal emission

      c. Manipulations: Gun, An, Rou, and Yizhichan Tui

21. Zhishi (BL 52)

      a. Location: 1.5 *cun* lateral to Shenshu (BL 23)

      b. Indications: Nocturnal emission, impotence, irregular menstruation, enuresis, and chronic lumbago

      c. Manipulations: Gun, Rou, An, and Yizhichan Tui

22. Chengshan (BL 57)

      a. Location: the top of the depression between both bellies of *m. gastrocnemius*

      b. Indication: Pain in the loins and legs, systremma, and diarrhea

      c. Manipulations: Gun, An, Rou, Na, and Ca

23. Kunlun (BL 60)

      a. Location: In the depression between the lateral malleolus and the Achilles tendon

      b. Indications: Headache, rigidity of the neck, lumbago, and sprained ankle

      c. Manipulations: An, Na, and DiAn

3.3.8. THE KIDNEY CHANNEL OF FOOT-SHAOYIN

This channel starts from the inferior aspect of the small toe, goes obliquely towards Yongquan (KI 1) in the center of the sole, emerges from the lower aspect of the tuberosity of the navicular bone, travels behind the medial malleolus and reaches the heel, ascends along the medio-posterior aspect of the shank, the popliteal fossa and the thigh, and enters the vertebral column, ascends further in the column, arrives at the kidney—the organ to which it belongs—and connects with the urinary bladder, and re-emerges from the pubic bone, runs upward through the abdomen, and ends at Shufu (KI 27) below the clavicle of the thorax.

The branch from the kidney runs straight up through the liver and the diaphragm, enters the lung, ascends along the throat, and terminates at both sides of the root of the tongue.

The branch from the lung joins the heart and runs into the chest to link with the Pericardium Channel of Hand-Hueyin.

The Kidney Channel of Foot-Shaoyin is exteriorly-interiorly related to the Bladder Channel. Along both routes of it, there are 54 points, of which the following are commonly used (See Figure 20).

1. Yongquan (KI1)

    a. Location: On the sole, in the depression when the foot is in plantar flexion

    b. Indications: Migraine, hypertension, infantile fever, vomiting, diarrhea, and insomnia

    c. Manipulations: Ca, An, Rou, and Na

2. Zhaohai (KI 6)

    a. Location: In the depression on the lower border of the medial malleolus

    b. Indications: Irregular menstruation, pain in the lower abdomen, dry throat, aphasia, and retention of urine

    c. Manipulations: An and Rou

3.3.9. THE PERICARDIUM CHANNEL OF HAND-JUEYIN

This channel originates in the chest, enters the pericardium—the organ to which it belongs—and after emerging, descends through the diaphragm, and passes the abdomen to connect successively with the upper-, middle- and lower-*jiao*.

The branch arising from the chest runs inside the chest, comes out from Tianchi (PC 1) in the costal region, travels transversely to the axillary

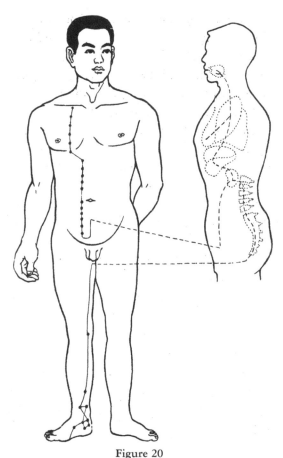

Figure 20

fold, descends into the palm along the middle line of the medial side of the upper arm and between the tendons of *m. palmaris longus* and *m. flexocarpi* of the forearm, and passes along the middle finger up to the tip where Zhongchong (PC 9) is located.

The branch arising from the palm leaves Laogong (PC 8) and runs along the ring finger up to the tip where it connects with the Sanjiao Channel of Hand-Shaoyang.

The Pericardium Channel of Hand-Jueyin is exteriorly-interiorly related to the Sanjiao Channel. Along both routes of it, there are 18 points. The commonly used ones are as follows (See Figure 21).

1. Quze (PC 3)

   a. Location: On the transverse cubital crease, at the ulnar side of the tendon of *m. biceps brachii*.

   b. Indications: Angina pectoris and soreness and tremor of the arm

   c. Manipulations: Na, An, and Rou

2. Neiguan (PC 6)

   a. Location: 2 *cun* above the transverse crease of the wrist, between the tendons of *m. palmaris longus* and *m. flexor radialis*

   b. Indications: Stomachache, vomiting, palpitation, angina pectoris hypertension, asthma, and mental disease

   c. Manipulations: Yizhichan Tui, An, Rou, and Na

3. Laogong (PC 8)

   a. Location: on the transverse crease of the palm, between the 2nd and 3rd metacarpal bones

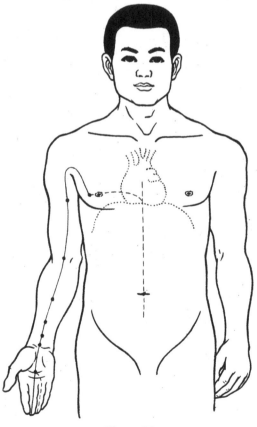

Figure 21

b. Indications: Psychosis, palpitation, heatstroke, and vomiting

c. Manipulations: An, Qia, and Na

4. Zhongchong (PC 9)

a. Location: At the tip of the middle finger

b. Indications: Coma, fever, heatstroke, and difficulty in speaking due to a stiff tongue

c. Manipulations: Qia and Qiarou

3.3.10. THE SANJIAO CHANNEL OF HAND-SHAOYANG

This channel starts from the point of Guanchong (SJ 1) at the tip of the ring finger, runs upward to the shoulder from between the 4th and 5th metacarpal bones and then between the radius and the ulna of the forearm, via the olecranon and along the lateral aspect of the upper arm, and finally goes forward from the shoulder to the supraclavicular fossa. From the fossa, it comes down into the chest and spreads there, connecting with the pericardium. Descending and passing through the diaphragm, it enters in succession the three *jiao* in the stomach—the organ to which it pertains.

The branch arising from the chest ascends, comes out of the same supraclavicular fossa, ascends to the neck, runs long the posterior border of the ear, winds to the anterior border of the ear, descends along the temple to the cheek, and terminates in the infraorbital region.

The branch arising from the retroauricular region enters the ear. Then it emerges in front of the ear, crosses the previous branch at the cheek and reaches the outer canthus where Sizhukong (SJ 23) is located, linking with the Gallbladder Channel of Foot-Shaoyang.

The Sanjiao Channel of Hand-Shaoyang has the exterior-interior relationship with the Pericardium Channel. Along both routes of it, there are 46 points altogether. The following are the commonly used ones (See Figure 22).

1. Zhongzhu (SJ 3)

a. Location: When the fist is naturally clenched, the point is on the dorsum of the hand, in the depression between the posterior borders of the small ends of the 4th and 5th metacarpal bones

b. Indication: Migraine, pain in the palm and finger with difficulty in flexion and extension, and pain in the elbow and arm

c. Manipulations: Rou and Yizhichan Tui

2. Waiguan (SJ 5)

a. Location: 2 *cun* above the dorsal carpal transverse crease between the radius and the ulna

b. Indications: Headache, pain, and motor impairment of the elbow, arm, and finger

c. Manipulations: Yizhichan Tui, Qia, An, and Rou

3. Jianliao (SJ 14)

a. Location: Lateral and inferior to the acromion, in the depression about 1 *cun* posterior to the point Jianyu (LI 15)

b. Indications: Soreness of the shoulder and arm and motor impairment of the shoulder

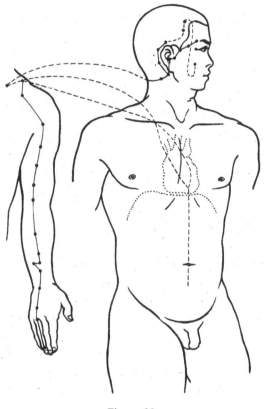

Figure 22

c. Manipulations: Yizhichan Tui, An, Rou, Gun, and Na

3.3.11. THE GALLBLADDER CHANNEL OF FOOT-SHAOYANG

This channel originates from the outer canthus where the point Tongziliao (GB 1) is located, ascends to the temple, curves downward to the retroauricular region, descends along the side of the neck to the shoulder, and enters the supraclavicular fossa.

The retroauricular branch arises from retroauricular region and enters the ear. Then it emerges from the preauricular region and goes along to the posterior aspect of the outer canthus.

The branch arising from the outer canthus descends to Daying (ST 5) and meets the Sanjiao Channel of Hand-Shaoyang in the infraorbital region, goes downward to pass through Jiache (ST 6) and to arrive at the shoulder, enters the supraclavicular fossa where it meets the main channel, falls into the chest, travels through the diaphragm, connects with the liver, and enters the gallbladder—the organ to which it pertains. Then it runs downwards along the inner side of the hypochondrium, comes out of the groin, passes through the vulva, and goes transversely into the hip joint region.

The branch going down from the supraclavicular fossa passes in front of the axilla along the lateral aspect of the chest and hypochondrium to the hip region where it meets the previous branch. Then it descends along the lateral aspect of the thigh and knee, the anterior aspect of the fibula and the anterior aspect of the lateral malleolus. It ends the lateral side of the tip of the 4th toe where the point Zuqiaoyin (GB 44) is located.

The branch starting from the dorsum of the foot connects with the Liver Channel of Foot-Jueyin.

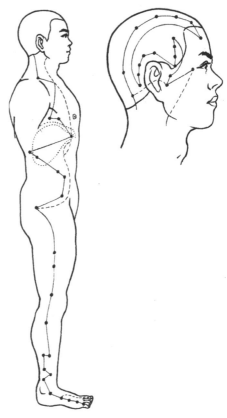

Figure 23

The Gallbladder Channel of Foot-Shaoyang is exteriorly-interiorly related to the Liver Channel. Along both routes of it, there are 88 points altogether. The following ones are commonly used (See Figure 23).

1. Tongziliao (GB 1)

   a. Location: Lateral to the outer canthus, on the lateral border of the orbital bone

   b. Indications: Migraine, conjunctivitis, myopia, and optic atrophy

   c. Manipulations: Rou, An, and Yizhichan Tui

2. Yangbai (GB 14)

   a. Location: When looking is directed straight ahead, the point is 1 *cun* directly above the midpoint of the eyebrow

   b. Indications: Facial paralysis, headache, and prosopalgia

   c. Manipulations: An, Mo, Pianfengtui, and Rou

3. Fengchi (GB 20)

   a. Location: Between the sternocleidomastoid muscle and the trapezial muscle, at the same level of Fengu (DU 16)

   b. Indications: Migraine, headache, common cold, neurosism, mental disease, rigidity of the neck, myopia, and hypertension

   c. Manipulations: Yizhichan Tui, An, Rou, DiAn, and Na

4. Jianjing (GB 21)

   a. Location: On the midway between Dazhui (DU 14) and the acromion and at the highest point of the shoulder

   b. Indications: Rigidity of the neck, soreness of the shoulder and back, mastitis, and motor impairment of the arm

   c. Manipulations: Na, Rou, Yizhichan Tui, and Gun

5. Juliao (GB 29)

   a. Location: On the midway between the anterosuperior iliac spine and the great trochanter of femur

   b. Indications: Pain in the loins and legs, soreness of the hip joint, sacro-illius, and inflammation of the superior clunial nerves

   c. Manipulations: Gun, An, DiAn, and Ya

6. Huantiao (GB 30)

   a. Location: At the junction of the lateral one-third and medial two-thirds of the distance between the great trochanter of femur and the hiatus of sacrum

   b. Indications: Pain in the loins and legs and paralysis of the lower extremities

   c. Manipulations: Gun, DiAn, An, and Ya

7. Fengshi (GB 31)

   a. Location: On the midline of the lateral aspect of the thigh, 7 *cun* above the transverse popliteal crease

   b. Indications: Paralysis of the lower extremities, soreness of the knee, and inflammation of the lateral cutaneous nerve of the thigh

   c. Manipulations: Gun, DiAn, An, and Ca

8. Yanglingquan (GB 34)

   a. Location: In the depression anterior and inferior to the small end of the fibula

   b. Indications: Painful knee, hypochondriac pain, paralysis of the legs, and cholecystitis

c. Manipulations: Na, DiAn, An, and Rou

9. Xuanzhong (GB 39)

   a. Location: 3 *cun* above the tip of the lateral malleolus, on the anterior border of the fibula

   b. Indications: Headache, rigidity of the neck, soreness of the legs, paralysis, and ankle disorders

   c. Manipulations: Na, DiAn, An, and Rou

10. Xiuxu (BG 40)

   a. Location: Anterior and inferior to the lateral malleolus, in the depression on the lateral side of the tendon of *m. extensordigitorum longus*

   b. Indications: Ankle pain, leg paralysis, and chest and hypochondriac pain.

   c. Manipulations: An, DiAn, Na, and Rou

3.3.12. THE LIVER CHANNEL OF FOOT-JUEYIN

This channel originates from the point Dadun (LR 1) at the tip of the big toe, runs upward along the dorsum of the foot, the anterior border of the medial malleols and the medial aspects of the shank, the knee and the thigh to the pubic hair region, curves around the external genitalia, and goes upward to the lower abdomen. From there it divides into two. One goes obliquely to the point Qimen (LR 14) between both ribs inferior to the nipple. The other runs upward and curves around the stomach to enter the liver—the organ to which it belongs—and connects with the gallbladder. Then it continues to ascend, passing through the diaphragm and branching out in the chest and hypochondriac region. Further upward, it reaches the nasopharynx region along the posterior aspect of the throat, connecting with the eye system. Finally, it ascends along the forehead to meet the Du Channel at the vertex.

The branch arising from the eye system runs downward into the cheek and curves around the inner surface of the lips.

The branch arising from the liver goes upward to pass the diaphragm, enters the lung and links with the Lung Channel of Hand-Taiyin.

The Liver Channel of Foot-Jueyin is exteriorly-interiorly related to the Gallbladder Channel. Along it, there are 28 points altogether, 14 on the left route, four on the right route. The commonly used ones are as follows (See Figure 24).

1. Taichong (LR 3)

   a. Location: On the dorsum of the foot, in the depression distal to the junction of the 1st and 2nd metatarsals

   b. Indications: Headache, vertigo, hypertension, hypochondriac pain, infantile convulsion, mental disease, and swelling and pain in the dorsum of the foot

   c. Manipulations: An, DiAn, Rou, and Yizhichan Tui

2. Zhangmen (LR 13)

   a. Location: At the free end of the 11th rib

   b. Indications: Distending pain in the chest and hypochondriac region, choking sensation in the chest, and cholecystitis

   c. Manipulations: An, Rou, and Mo

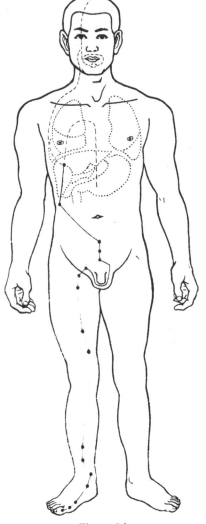

Figure 24

3.3.13. THE REN CHANNEL

This channel originates in the lower abdomen and emerges from the perineum. It goes straight upward to the throat along the midline of the abdomen and chest. From there, it ascends to the point Chengjiang (RN 24). Ascending further, it curves around the lips, passes the cheek, and enters the infraorbital region. (See Figure 25). Along it, there are 24 points altogether. The commonly used ones are as follows.

1. Qugu (RN 2)

   a. Location: On the midline of the abdomen and on the upper border of the symphysis pubis

   b. Indications: Nocturnal emission, impotence, and retention of urine

   c. Manipulations: An, DiAn, and Rou

2. Zhongji (RN 3)

   a. Location: On the midline of the abdomen, 4 *cun* below the umbilicus

   b. Indications: Pain in the lower abdomen, enuresis, retention of urine, irregular menstruation, and pelvic inflammation

   c. Manipulations: Yizhichan Tui, Mo, Rou, DiAn, and An

3. Guanyuan (RN 4)

   a. Location: 3 *cun* below the umbilicus

   b. Indications: Irregular menstruation, dysmenorrhea, nocturnal emission, impotence, enuresis, and chronic diarrhea

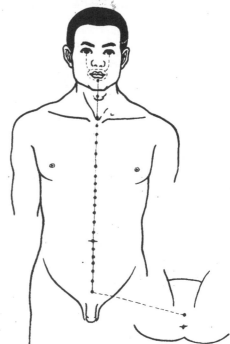

Figure 25

   c. Manipulations: Mo, Rou, An, DiAn, and Yizhichan Tui

4. Qihai (RN 6)

   a. Location: 1.5 *cun* below the umbilicus

   b. Indications: Noctural emission, impotence, dysmenorrhea, diarrhea, enuresis, and irregular menstruation

   c. Manipulations: Mo, An, Rou, and Zhen

5. Zhongwan (RN 12)

   a. Location: 4 *cun* above the umbilicus

   b. Indications: Stomachache, abdominal distension, vomiting, and indigestion

   c. Manipulations: Mo, An, Rou, and Zhen

6. Danzhong (RN 17)

   a. Location: On the midline of the abdomen, at the level of the 4th intercostal space

   b. Indications: Cough and asthma, stuffiness and pain in the chest, hiccups, mastitis, and angina pectoris

   c. Manipulations: Yizhichan Tui, Mo, An, and Rou

7. Tiantu (RN 22)

   a. Location: At the center of the suprasternal fossa

   b. Indications: Cough with dyspnea, difficulty in coughing up sputum, aphasia, and hiccups

   c. Manipulations: Rou, An, Qia, and DiAn

8. Lianquan (RN 23)

   a. Location: Above the Adam's apple, in the depression of the upper border of the hyoid bone

   b. Indications: Aphasia, stiff tongue, difficulty in swallowing, and laryngopharyngitis

   c. Manipulations: An, Rou, DiAn, and Tanbo

9. Chengjiang (RN 24)

   a. Location: In the center of the mentolabial sulcus

   b. Indication: Facial paralysis, prosopalgia, and toothache

   c. Manipulations: An, Rou, and Qia

3.3.14. THE DU CHANNEL

This channel starts from in the lower abdomen and emerges from the perineum, and then goes backwards to the point Changqiang (DU 1). From there, it runs upward along the interior of the spinal column all the way, passing Fengfu (DU 16), entering the brain and reaching the vertex. Going further, it winds along the forehead to the columnella of the nose, passes the point Renzhong (DU 26) or the groove of the upper lip, and ends at the point Yinjiao (DU 28) at the upper labial frenum (See Figure 26). Along this channel, there are 28 points, of which the following are commonly used.

1. Changqiang (DU 1)

   a. Location: 0.5 *cun* interior to the tip of the coccyx

   b. Indications: Diarrhea, constipation, prolapse of the rectum, and pain in the waist and spine

   c. Manipulations: Rou and An

2. Yaoyangguan (DU 3)

   a. Location: Below the spinous process of the 4th lumbar vertebra

   b. Indications: Pain in the loins and spine and paralysis of the legs

   c. Manipulations: Gun, Uizhichan Tui, An, Rou, and Ca

3. Mingmen (DU 4)

  a. Location: Below the spinous process of the 2nd lumbar vertebra

  b. Indications: Pain in the waist and spine, noctural emission, impotence, chronic diarrhea, irregular menstruation, and dysmenorrhea

  c. Manipulations: Gun, Yizhichan Tui, An, Rou, and Ca

4. Shenzhu (DU 12)

  a. Location: Below the spinous process of the 3rd thoracic vertebra

  b. Indications: Cough and backache

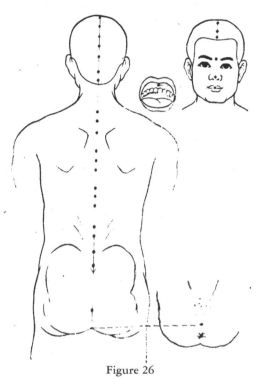

Figure 26

  c. Manipulations: Gun, An, Rou, and Yizhichan Tui

5. Dazhui (DU 14)

  a. Location: Below the spinous process of the 7th cervical vertebra

  b. Indications: Common cold, fever, stiff neck, cough, asthma, and pain in the neck and back

  c. Manipulations: Gun, An, Rou, and Yizhichan Tui

6. Fengfu (DU 16)

  a. Location: 1 *cun* directly above the midpoint of the posterior hairline

  b. Indications: Neck rigidity, mental disorders, and apoplexy

  c. Manipulations: Yizhichan Tui, An, Rou, and DiAn

7. Baihui (DU 20)

  a. Location: 7 *cun* directly above the posterior hairline, on the midpoint of the line connecting the apexes of both auricles

  b. Indications: Headache, dizziness, coma, hypertension, prolapse of the rectum, and mental disorders

c. Manipulations: An, Rou, Yizhichan Tui, and Zhen

8. Shuigou, also called as Renzhong (DU 26)

   a. Location: At the junction of the upper one-third and the lower two-thirds of the midline of the nasolabial groove

   b. Indications: Infantile convulsion, facial paralysis, mental disorders, and acute sprained wrist

   c. Manipulations: Qia and Rou

3.4 Other Points Commonly Used in Tuina Manipulations

1. Yintang (EX-HN 3)

   a. Location: At the midpoint between the medial ends of both eyebrows

   b. Indications: Headache, rhinitis, and insomnia

   c. Manipulations: Yizhichan Tui, Mo, An, and Rou

2. Taiyang (EX-S/HE 5)

   a. Location: In the depression about 1 *cun* posterior to the midpoint between the lateral end of the eyebrow and the outer canthus

   b. Indications: Headache, common cold, and eye disease

   c. Manipulations: An, Rou, Mo, and Yizhichan Tui

3. Yuyao (EX-HN 4)

   a. Location: At the midpoint of the eyebrow

   b. Indications: Pain in the supraorbital region, redness, swelling and pain of the eyes, and twitching of the eyelids

   c. Manipulations: Mo, Yizhichan Tui, and An

4. Yaoyan (EX-B 7)

   a. Location: In the depression 3 *cun* lateral to the inferior border of the spinous process of the 3rd lumbar vertebra

   b. Indications: Lumbar sprain and aching of the loins

   c. Manipulations: Gun, An, Na, and Ca

5. Jaiji (EX-B 2)

   a. Location: on the line 0.5 *cun* lateral to the inferior border of each spinous process from the 1st thoracic vertebra to the 5th lumbar vertebra

   b. Indications: Pain and stiffness in the spinal column and diseases of the internal organs

  c. Manipulations: Gun, Ca, Ya, Tui, and Yizhichan Tui

6. Shiqizhui (EX-B 8)

  a. Location: Below the spinous process of the 5th lumbar vertebra

  b. Indications: Pain in the loins and legs and dysmenorrhea

  c. Manipulations: DiAn, Gun, and An

7. Shixuan (EX-UE 11)

  a. Location: At the tip of each of the ten fingers, 0.1 *cun* away from the nail

  b. Indications: Coma

  c. Manipulations: Qia

8. Heding (EX-LE 2)

  a. Location: In the depression at the center of the upper border of the patella

  b. Indications: Swelling and pain in the knee

  c. Manipulations: An, Rou, and DiAn

9. Lanwei (EX-LE 7)

  a. Location: About 2 *cun* below the point Zusanli (ST 36)

  b. Indications: Appendicitis and abdominal pain

  c. Manipulations: An, Rou, and DiAn

10. Jianneiling

  a. Location: At the midpoint of the line connecting the tip of the anterior axillary fold and the point Jianyu (LI 15)

  b. Indications: Pain and motor impairment of the shoulder

  c. Manipulations: Yizhichan Tui, Gun, Na, An, and Rou

11. Qiaogong

  a. Location: along the line between the inferior and anterior of the temporal process and the point Quepen (ST 12) at the supraclavicular fossa

  b. Indications: Headache, dizziness, and hypertension

  c. Manipulations: Pushing downward with the thumb

CHAPTER 4

Common Tuina
Manipulations

Manipulation refers to the way that a practitioner performs standardized technical maneuvers on the joints, along the channels, and over the specific portion of a patient's body for medical purposes. Manipulation is the primary means that tuina is used to treat diseases. Good curative effects come from good clinical choice and performance of manipulations.

Ancient and modern medical specialists have created many effective tuina manipulations, more than 110 of which are recorded in written language. However, no more than 20 or 30 of them are commonly used. Each manipulation is undertaken according to its own pattern of standardized technical movements. This pattern is called the makeup of movement, which mainly includes the following factors:

- The posture of the whole body
- Breathing
- Preparatory gesture of manipulation movement
- Stage of movement
- Essentials of movement
- Angle, amplitude, frequency, rhythm, and periodicity of each movement
- Work and interrelation of different acting muscles

The manipulating techniques of traditional tuina medicine are basically characterized by permanence, forcefulness, evenness, and softness, all of which combine to produce a deepening effect.

Permanence. Manipulations are performed for a certain required time during which the manipulation should remain the same in its makeup or in its dynamic pattern.

Forcefulness. Manipulations exert a certain power, and the volume should be changed according to the patient's constitution, disease, and age, and according to the manipulated part as well.

Evenness. Manipulations should be rhythmic with constant frequency and pressure.

Softness. Manipulations should be gentle but not superficial, heavy but not sluggish, powerful but not rough or violent, and smooth with its maneuvers changing naturally

Deepening. Manipulations should be performed with the direction of its acting force properly adjusted so that the effect of the applied dynamic force may go deep into the body and act on the target tissue where the disorder is located.

Of course, all the above factors are closely and organically interrelated; together, they are the technical essentials of every maneuver of every kind of tuina manipulation. Manipulations are different in the makeup of each maneuver, so they are also different in technique. For instance, the manipulations of Yi Zhi Chan Tui Fa (operated with one thumb) and Gun Fa (rolling) are firm but primarily gentle. On the other hand, Ji DiAn Fa (digital hitting) is accurate, resolute, rapid, and gentle but primarily firm. Mo is slow, gentle or strong, but primarily moderate. In the course of training in manipulation techniques, it is important to study the features unique to any manipulation in order to master the techniques.

The following is an introduction to 20 commonly used manipulations and the methods for mastering them through training.

4.1 Yizhichan Tui (work with one thumb)

Explanation. Put the lateral surface of the thumb's tip on the part to be operated. Relax the shoulder, drop the elbow, and raise the wrist. Flex and stretch the elbow cyclically and swing the forearm inward and outward so as to bring about the flexion and extension of the thumb joint (See Figure 27).

Essentials. Cup the fist by flexing naturally—but not closing tightly—the index, middle, ring and little fingers. Cover the fist hole with the thumb. Relax the muscles of the arm. Exert acting force naturally and avoid forceful pressure after the thumb is fixed on the operated point. Keep steady pressure, frequency, and amplitude of swing so that the produced force can act on the part being treated rhythmically and continuously. The frequency of this manipulation should be between 120-160 times per minute.

Application. This manipulation is characterized by a small force-bearing point; great pressure intensity; a strong deepening effect;

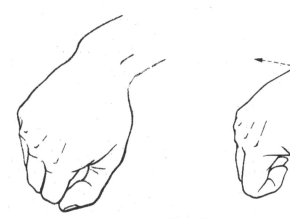

Figure 27

continuous, rhythmic, and gentle stimula given to the patient; and stimulation volume regulated as needed. It may be performed everywhere on the body, including on the channels, points, and other parts. It is used to treat common diseases of medicine, surgery, trauma, gynecology, and the five sense organs.

Variations.

1. Pressing with the lateral surface of the thumb is called Luowen Tui. This variation is especially suitable for performance on the abdomen and chest and for treating diseases of the digestive system and female reproductive system

2. Pressing with the tip of the thumb is called Zhongfeng Tui. This variation is most effective in treating diseases of medicine such as headache, dizziness, insomnia, hypertension, and disorder due to stagnation of the liver-qi

3. Pressing with the very tip of the thumb is called Chanfa. This variation is smaller in amplitude of the swing. It is performed at a faster rhythm (200-240 times per minute). Chanfa creates unique curative effects when used to treat laryngological diseases and surgical carbuncle and furuncle

4. Pressing with the side of the thumb radius is called Pianfeng Tui. This variation is suitable for the craniofacial region and is often used to treat myopia, rhinorrhea with turbid discharge, stuffy or running nose, headache, distending sensation in the head, tinnitus, facial paralysis, prosopalgia, and toothache.

4.2 Na (grasp)

Explanation. The thumb and the index and middle fingers—or the thumb and the other four fingers—exert slow and symmetrical forces to hold and pull and simultaneously twist and knead the treated part, which is then released. This maneuver is repeated again and again (See Figure 28).

Essentials. Stretch each interphalangeal joint of the thumb and the other four fingers and do the work with finger surfaces. Do not flex the fingers lest you dig the treated part with fingernails. Ensure harmonious and rhythmical movements of the wrist and finger joints. Add force slowly and gently when pulling until it optimal. Avoid a sudden decrease or increase of the force, as well as sudden holding and releasing of the part with violent force.

Application. This manipulation produces strong stimulation that, in the short run, will make the patient feel strongly sore and distending. It is often applied to the cord-like soft tissues such as muscles and tendons of the neck, shoulder, back, lateral abdomen, and limbs. It is used to:

- Induce resuscitation and restore consciousness
- Relieve superficies syndrome by means of diaphoresis
- Expel wind and clear away cold
- Relax muscles and tendons to promote blood circulation
- Relieve spasm and pain

When performed in clinical practice, the practitioner can use either one hand or two. The decision is based on the treated part and the disease being treated.

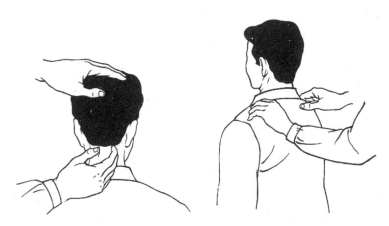

Figure 28

4.3 An (press)

Explanation. With finger or palm, press the operated part vertically: with each press, start slowly, gently, and superficially and then proceed forcefully and deeply until the specific depth is reached. Press for five to ten seconds. When you stop pressing, leave the finger or palm on the operated part, then slowly take away the finger or palm. Repeat as prescribed.

Essentials. Breathe naturally during the entire manipulation and do not hold back breath when emitting force. Exert force steadily, a little less at the beginning, and gradually more and more until the patient experiences soreness, distension, numbness, and/or radiation.

When more powerful and repeated operations are needed, the best way to save strength and affect good results is as follows: Stretch both arms straight; put one thumb or one palm on the other and press the operated part one time after another. Each time, lean your body slightly forward as if you are supporting it on the operated part with your arms. This way, your body weight is utilized instead of the force exerted actively by the fingers or arms.

Applications. An is a manipulation whose stimulation should be changed from mild degree to moderate one. It should be performed until the patient has got the above-mentioned sensations. Pressing with the fingers may be conducted on the points of all parts of the body, while pressing with the palm, on the loins, back and abdomen.

Variations.
1. Pressing with the thumb is called Muzhi An.
2. Pressing with the middle finger is Zhongzhi An.

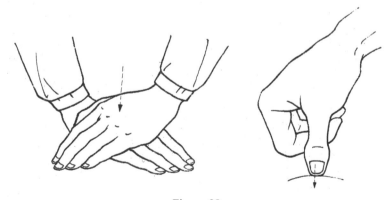

Figure 29

3. Pressing with the palm is Zhang An.

4. Pressing digitally is DianAn-An.

5. Pressing with the palm base is Zhanggen An (Figure 29).

4.4 Mo (palm rub)

Explanation. Rhythmically rub the treated part with the palm or the palmar sides of the index, middle, ring, and small fingers. Rub in a circle, clockwise or counterclockwise.

Essentials. The acting force is gentle and mild, the rhythm is steady, and the frequency is moderate, usually about 100-200 circles per minute.

Application. As one of the commonly used manipulations of tuina, this manipulation is mainly applicable to the chest, hypochondrium, epigastrium, and abdomen. It is often used to treat epigastric and abdominal pain, distension due to stagnant food, choking sensation in the chest due to stagnation of *qi*, and impairment of the chest and hypochondrium. Its action relieves the depressed liver and promotes the *qi* flow, warms the middle-*jiao* and normalizes the function of the stomach, removes retained food, and regulates gastrointestinal peristalsis.

Variations.

1. Rubbing with the palm is called Zhang Mo

2. Rubbing with the surface of the four fingers (and not the thumb) is called Zhi Mo (See Figure 30).

4.5 Rou (knead)

Explanation. Gently and slowly knead and rotate the treated part with the fingers, palm base, and major thenar.

Essentials. Put the finger, palm base, or major thenar on the treated part and knead the skin in a small circle. Use your whole body for this; coordinate the movements of the shoulder, elbow, forearm, and wrist so that gentle and slow internal friction is caused between the skin and the soft tissue beneath it. The kneading must be gentle, but as the circle becomes gradually larger, the force grows step by step. Make sure that the operating part is fixed on the treated part lest friction and slipping occur between the operating part and the skin of the treated part. Proper kneading frequency is 100-140 times per minute.

Application. Rou may be used all over the body. It soothes the oppressed chest, regulates the *qi* flow, strengthens the spleen, normalizes the function of the stomach, promotes blood circulation, removes blood stasis, relieves swelling, stops pain, and tranquilizes the mind. It is often used to treat headaches, vertigo, facial paralysis, distending pain in the epigastric and abdominal regions, choking sensation in the chest, hypochondriac pain, constipation, diarrhea, and swelling and pain of soft tissue due to trauma.

Variations.

1. Kneading with the middle finger is called Zhongzhi Rou. It is applied to the channels and points all over the body and areas where digital stimulation is needed.

2. Kneading with the thumb is Muzhi Rou. Like Zhongzhi, it is applied to the channels and points all over the body and areas where digital stimulation is needed.

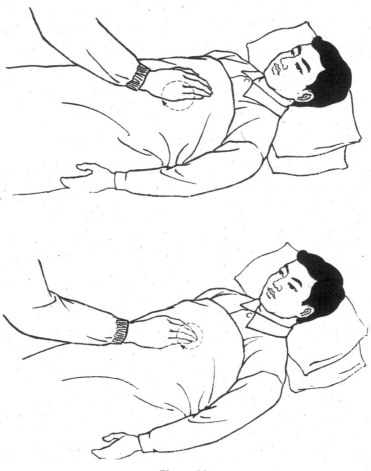

Figure 30

3. Kneading with the palm base is Zhanggen Rou. It is applied to the back, loins, buttock, and thick muscles of the limbs

4. Kneading with the major thenar is Dayuji Rou. This manipulation is applicable to the craniofacial area, the thoracia-abdominal region, and sprained limbs.

5. Kneading with the elbow is Zhou Rou (See Figure 31). Zhou Rou is applied to the deep layer of tissue.

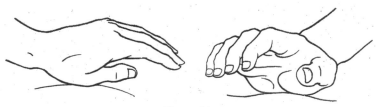

Figure 31

4.6 DiAn (digital press)

Explanation. More forceful and vertical than An, DiAn is the operated with the very tip of the thumb or the middle finger or with the flexed, protruded, and proximal interphalangeal joint of the middle or index finger or the thumb.

Essentials. Breathe naturally and avoid holding your breath when pressing. Begin with light and superficial force and gradually add heavy and deepening force. The force exerted should be strong enough to make the patient have strong sensations of soreness, distention, and/or numbness, but these sensations should be within the range that the patient can handle. Avoid applying too much force lest ecchymoma occur or unbearable sufferings be brought to the patient.

Application. DiAn is a digital-striking manipulation with strong stimulation. Its acting points are small and concentrating, its effect is deepening like what is induced by acupuncture. Therefore, it is often used to strike the mass or pressure pain point that is deep in the muscles or between the bones. It is designed to make the patient strongly feel sore, numb, distended and/or pain, thus stopping pain by the induced pain. This manipulation is usually applied to the treatment of epigastric and abdominal pain due to spasm, pain of the limbs due to pertinacious stagnation of *qi* and blood or old injury, and numbness and paralysis.

Variations.

1. Pressing with the tip of the middle finger is called Zhongzhi DiAn.

2. Pressing with the tip of the thumb is Muzhi DiAn.

3. Pressing with an interphalangeal joint is Zhijie DiAn (See Figure 32).

4.7 Ca (rub)

Explanation. Rub the treated part to and fro in a straight direction with the palm, minor thenar or major thenar.

Essentials. Ca requires a large amplitude, a distance as long as possible, and a straight direction no matter how it may be done on the surface of the body: straight upward and downward, across from left to right, or obliquely. In addition, keep the operating hand touching the

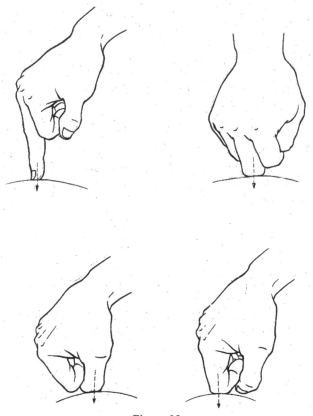

Figure 32

skin of the treated. The acting force should be always even along the whole trail of Ca. Meanwhile, the force should be moderate, for rubbing with hard pressure tends to injure the skin.

Application. Ca and Mo are the same in rubbing but they are different in the following: the former is done in a straight direction, while the latter, in a circle, and the former is more powerful and produces more of a warming effect than the latter. Clinically, the more powerful and warming effect of Ca contributes to the following curative effects: warming the channels and alleviating pain, expelling wind and dispelling cold, relieving swelling and resolving mass, regulating the *qi* flow, and promoting blood circulation. When performed clinically conducted, attention should be paid to the following:

- Full exposure of the operated part
- One or two times of gentle and slow rubbing at the beginning followed by more rapid ones performed until local heat occurs
- Ten times of rubbing is usually enough for each treatment
- Prolonged performance is not advocated lest blisters occur on the skin due to overheating

In order to further protect the skin from being hurt and to help produce heat, use a medium—such as sesame oil, ointment of Chinese Holly Leaf, or Massage Emulsion— when performing this manipulation.

Variations.
1. Rubbing with the palm is called Zhang Ca.
2. Rubbing with the minor thenar is Xiaoyiji Ca.
3. Rubbing with the major thenar is Dayuji Ca (See Figure 33).

4.8 Gun (roll)

Explanation. Rotate the forearm outward and inward cyclically to lead to the flexion and extension of the wrist. This motion makes 1/3 to 1/2 of the slightly arched dorso-ulnar roll back and forth on the treated part (See Figure 34).

Essentials. The hand touches the skin of the treated part; avoid rubbing and sliding. The pressure is even, gentle, and constant; too powerful a push is avoided. Position yourself as follows:

- Keep forearm between prone 45 and supine 45.
- Keep the wrist between 45 when flexed and 10 when stretched.
- Flex the hand naturally without any active closing and extending.
- Relax the shoulder; let it naturally drop.

- Adjust the shoulder to 30 to 40 anteflexion and 30 abduction.
- Adjust the elbow to 90 to 120 flexed naturally.
- Perform between 140 to 160 times per minute.

Application. This manipulation involves a large area, produces powerful acting force, and is quite deepening in its effect. Except the craniofacial, anterior-cervical, and thoracico-abdominal regions, it can be applied on all parts of the body, especially on the loins, the back, the buttock and the thick muscles of the limbs. If the area of the second,

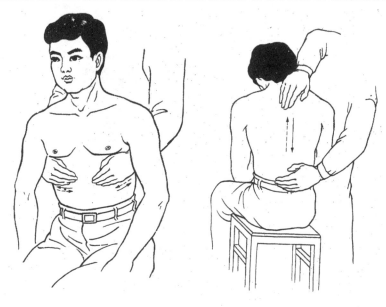

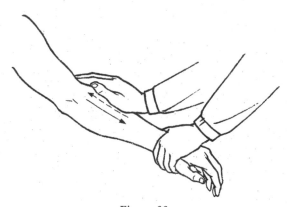

Figure 33

third, fourth, and fifth metacarpophalangeal joints is made to act on the treated part through regulating the posture of the hand, greater stimulation quantity will be produced. Gun has the following effects:

- Relaxes muscles and tendons and activates collaterals
- Expels wind and disperses cold
- Warms channels and removes dampness

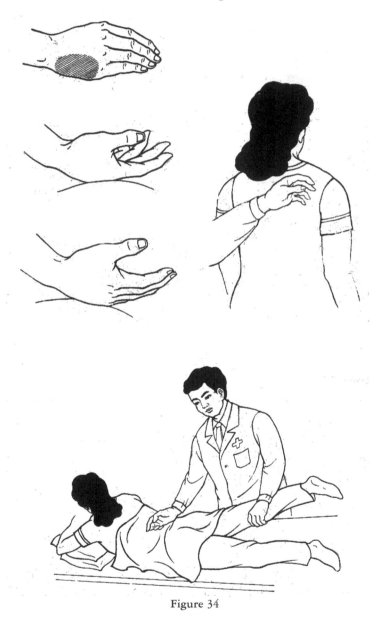

Figure 34

- Promotes blood circulation to dispel blood stasis
- Relieves spasm and stops pain
- Weakens adhesion and lubricates joints

As one of the most-often used manipulations in clinical practice, it is especially suitable for the treatment of disorders of the motor and nervous systems.

4.9 Zhen (vibrate)

Explanation. Put the tip of the middle finger or the palm on the treated part. Alternately contract the extensor and flexor muscles of the forearm. Do so rapidly and in a minor range so that gentle and constant vibration is produced. The vibration acts on the body through the tip of the middle finger or the palm on the treated part (See Figure 35).

Essentials. Do not forcefully press on the treated part or hold your breath to exert the force. The contraction of the muscles of the forearm causes the hand to produce vertical vibration. The frequency of the vibration is between 8-12 times per second. Make sure that the vibration is produced by the force; the force is directed by *qi*, and the *qi* is guided by the mind. The whole process of the maneuver is natural, consistent, harmonious, and integrated. To accomplish this, the practitioner must

- Concentrate his/her mind
- Lead *qi* down to the Dantian
- Regulate even breathing
- Use his/her mind to move the *qi* along the inside of the palm to the point of Laogong (at the center of the palm) or to the tip of the middle finger so that it may direct the force there.

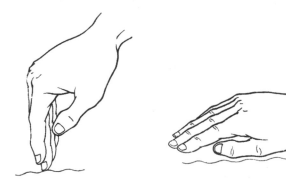

Figure 35

Application. Suitable for the application to all parts of the body, especially to the craniofacial and thoracico-abdominal regions, this manipulation may bring about such effects as tranquilizing the mind, improving eyesight, strengthening intelligence, warming up the middle-*jiao*, regulating the *qi* flow, promoting digestion, and adjusting enterogastric peristalsis. Therefore, better curative effects are achieved when Zhen is used to treat insomnia, amnesia, and gastrointestional dysfunction.

4.10 Cuo (foulage)

Explanation. Hold and then twist and rub the treated part of the body back and forth rapidly with both palms. The palms move upward and downward again and again at the same time (See Figure 36).

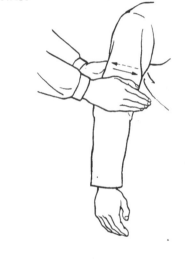

Essentials. The practitioner half-squats with his/her upper body leaning slightly forward and symmetrically applies force with both palms. Twists are rapid with even amplitude. The up-and-down motion of the palms is steady and slightly slow.

Application. Cuo is often performed over the upper torso and/or legs, the hypochondriac region, and/or the loins. Its effects are as follows:

- Regulates blood and *qi*
- Restores joints and tendons
- Relaxes muscles

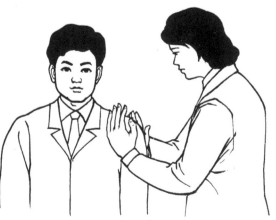

Figure 36

4.11 Mo (wipe)

Explanation. Rub the treated part in a straight direction, gently, vertically, or horizontally, and repeat with one or two thumbs. Touch the thumb(s) closely to the skin of the treated part while rubbing (See Figure 37).

Essentials. The force exerted should be moderate, because too much force blocks the movement and too little force keeps the movement on the surface. Apply with even frequency. When rubbing vertically, work with each thumb alternately. When rubbing horizontally, work both thumbs at the same time. Talcum powder may be used as a medium in summer when sweating tends to occur.

Application. Apply this manipulation to the craniofacial and cervical regions. It is usually used as the main or an auxiliary manipulation when dizziness, headache, facial paralysis, prosopalgia, and stiffness and pain of the nape are treated. It can play a part in inducing resuscitation, tranquilizing the mind, restoring consciousness, improving eyesight, relaxing muscles and tendons, and promoting blood circulation.

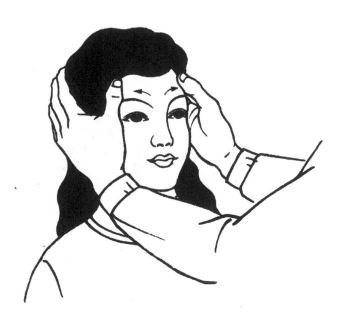

Figure 37

4.12 Tina (lift/grasp)

Explanation. The tendons or muscle bundles of a patient are held and lifted with the thumb, index, and middle fingers or with the thumb and the other four fingers (See Figure 38).

Essentials. This is a compound manipulation that combines lifting and holding. Its essentials are similar to those of Na, but its lift is more powerful.

Stretch each interphalangeal joint of the thumb and the other four fingers and do the work with finger surfaces. Do not flex the fingers lest you dig the treated part with fingernails. Ensure harmonious and rhythmical movements of the wrist and finger joints. Add force slowly and gently when pulling until it is optimal. Avoid a sudden decrease or increase of the force, as well as sudden holding and releasing of the part with violent force.

Application. This manipulation produces stronger stimulation. Tina excites nerves, activates *yang-qi*, removes stagnation, expels wind, and disperses cold. Evident curative effects are attained when used to treat myophagism, nerve paralysis, stubborn arthralgia due to wind-dampness, and hemiparalysis.

4.13 AnRou (press/knead)

Explanation. The manipulations of An and Rou are combined so that you are kneading while pressing.

Essentials. For the kneading portion of this manipulation, put the finger, palm base, or major thenar on the treated part and knead the

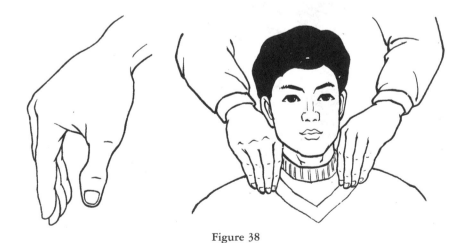

Figure 38

skin in a small circle. Use your whole body for this; coordinate the movements of the shoulder, elbow, forearm, and wrist so that gentle and slow internal friction is caused between the skin and the soft tissue beneath it. The kneading must be gentle, but as the circle becomes gradually larger, the force grows step by step. Make sure that the operating part is fixed on the treated part lest friction and slipping occur between the operating part and the skin of the treated part. Proper kneading frequency is 100-140 times per minute.

For the pressing portion of this manipulation, exert force steadily, a little less at the beginning, and gradually more and more until the patient experiences soreness, distension, numbness, and/or radiation.

When more powerful and repeated operations are needed, the best way to save strength and affect good results is as follows: Stretch both arms straight; put one thumb or one palm on the other and press the operated part one time after another. Each time, lean your body slightly forward as if you are supporting it on the operated part with your arms. This way, your body weight is utilized instead of the force exerted actively by the fingers or arms.

Breathe naturally during the entire manipulation and do not hold back breath when emitting force.

Application. Having forcefulness and gentleness combined together, this manipulation can produce a kind of heavy and forceful but gentle and comfortable stimulus. It tranquilizes the mind, removes stasis, resolves mass, and relieves spasm and pain.

Generally, AnRou is applicable to the channels and points or non-fixed points all over the body. Specifically:

- AnRou with three fingers is applied to the thoracico-abdominal region (See variations below).

- AnRou with both thumbs is applied to the loins or hips where there are thick muscles.

- AnRou with one finger is applied to the craniofacial region and the limbs.

Variations.
1. Performing with three fingers such as the index, middle, and ring fingers is called Sanzhi AnRou.
2. Performing with both thumbs—one pressed on the other, exerting combined force on the treated point—is called Shuangzhi AnRou. This is used when hard pressure is needed on the point.
3. Using the thumb and the middle and index fingers is Sanzhi AnRou.

73

4.14 Boyun (forearm knead)

Explanation. Rub or knead the treated part with the upper belly of the forearm: about 1/3 of the ulnar flexor muscle (See Figure 39).

Essentials.

1. Preparatory posture: Sit with the shoulder relaxed (not lifted); extend the upper arm naturally forward with the elbow flexed about 90 to 100, and keep the forearm fully in the pronator position with the palm downwards and the fingers free.

2. Performance: Rhythmically extend and flex the elbow within 90-160 so that the rubbing and kneading effect occurs on the treated part. While performing, the practitioner sits upright with his/her upper body inclined a little forward. Be sure not to lean the upper body too much lest the movement is blocked.

Application. Boyun allows for the treatment of a larger surface than when rubbing or kneading with fingers or the palm. It also allows for greater pressure to be exerted, thus providing a deepening effect. Boyun is applicable to the loins, back, hip, thigh, the abdominal region, and other areas where large surface needs rubbing or kneading. Better curative effects are obtained when used to treat sprain, contusion, lumbar intervertebral disc, and sciatica.

4.15 Ji (beat)

Explanation.
Rhythmically beat the treated part with the back of a fist, the palmar base, the palm, the minor thenar, the tip of a finger or a mulberry stick (See Figure 40).

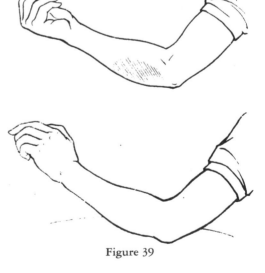

Essentials.

1. Beating with a fist. Cup the fist, extend the wrist straight, and beat the body surface with the back of the fist.

2. Beating with a palm. Flex the fingers

Figure 39

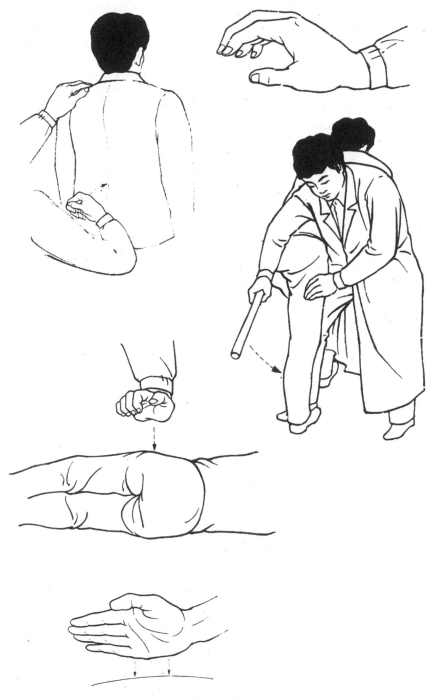

Figure 40

naturally, extend the wrist straight or a little backwards, and tap the treated part with the palm or palmar base.

3. Beating with the minor thenar (also called lateral beating or cutting beating). Extend the hand, palm, and wrist straight. Naturally abduct the thumb and close the other four fingers. Position the forearm and palm upright and beat the treated part rhythmically with the ulnar surface of the minor thenar. Alternate hands.

4. Beating with the fingers (also called digital beating or tapping). Beat the points on the body surface with the tip of the middle finger, the tips of the thumb, index and middle fingers, or the closed tips of all five fingers.

5. Beating with a stick. Beat the treated area of the body surface with a treating stick made of mulberry twigs.

Application.

1. Beating with the back of a fist is usually applied to the point of Dazhui and the lumbosacral portion.

2. Beating with the palm is applied to the anterior fontanelle of the vertex and the point of Baihui.

3. Beating with the minor thenar is applied to the lumbodorsal region and the limbs.

4. Beating with fingertip is applied to the channels and points of the head, face, chest, abdomen, and limbs.

5. Beating with a stick is applied to the vertex, shoulder, lumbosacral portion of the back, and limbs.

Ji relaxes the tendons and dredges the collaterals, promotes blood circulation to remove blood stasis, and regulates *qi* and blood. It treats arthralgia due to wind and dampness, numbness, muscular spasm, paralysis, and myophagism.

Process of Making Mulberry Stick. Strip the peel the 12 pieces of fresh mulberry twig, each of which is about 0.5 cm thick and dry them in the air. Roll each twig with mulberry paper, and then tightly coil each one with thread. Put the 12 pieces together and roll them again with mulberry paper round and round into a stick that is coiled with thread and wrapped with a piece of cloth. Finally sew the cloth well to complete. This stick, 4.5 cm to 5 cm in diameter and about 40 cm long, should be moderate in hardness and elasticity.

4.16 Pai (pat)

Explanation. Pat the body surface with a hollow palm (See Figure 41).

Essentials. Extend all five fingers with the 2nd, 3rd, 4th and 5th metacarpophalangeal joints slightly bent. This produces a concave palm called "hollow palm." Pat the treated part with the hollow palm. In doing so, the movement of the wrist follows that of the forearm so that the force exerted is elastic and skillful.

Application. This manipulation is mainly suitable for performance on the shoulder, back, lumbosacral portion, and thigh. Light patting may be conducted on the thoracico-abdominal region. Patting strongly for a long time tranquilizes and relieves pain, promotes blood circulation to remove blood stasis, alleviates spasm, and strengthens the body. Patting lightly for a short time clears away heat to benefit the mind, excites the nerves, regulates the intestines and stomach, soothes chest oppression, and activates the *qi* flow. Pai is often used to treat various kinds of arthralgia due to wind and dampness, overstrain due to old damage, blood stasis due to new injuries, myophagism, hypoesthesia, enteroparalysis, choking, painful sensation in the chest, and involuntary movement due to wrong exercise of *qigong*.

4.17 Dou (shake)

Explanation. Hold the distal end of an arm or a leg of a patient with both hands and shake it up and down. Be forceful and constant, but keep the range of motion small (See Figure 42).

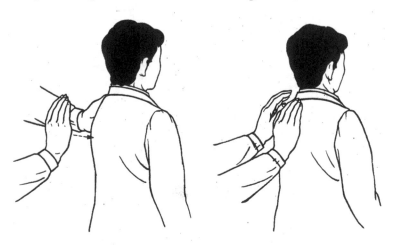

Figure 41

Essentials. Half-squat and lean the upper body slightly forward. Stretch both arms forward naturally with the elbow 130 to160 flexed. Hold the wrist or ankle with both hands and pull the operated limb straight. Fix the patient's arm in the abducted position of 45 to 60, or if treating a leg, raise the leg until a 30 angle is formed between it and the bed. Exert slow force to shake the operated limb up and down, constantly and narrowly. Do not squeeze the limb too tightly and do not pull the limb too much; keep the limb in a relaxed condition. The amplitude of shaking varies from small to moderate, and the frequency is rapid.

Application. Often combined with the manipulation of Cuo, this manipulation is usually used before a treatment is ended so as to relax the muscles and regulate the *qi* flow and blood in the limbs. Repeat ten times.

Variations. Dou is also used to shake the waist as follows: Raise, pull, and powerfully shake the patient's legs to cause the produced vibrating effect to reach the waist. Repeat three to four times. Dou is often used in this way to treat prolapse of lumbar intervertebral disc.

4.18 Yao (rotate)

Explanation. Hold the proximal end of the treated joint with one hand and the distal end with the other to cause the joint to do passive

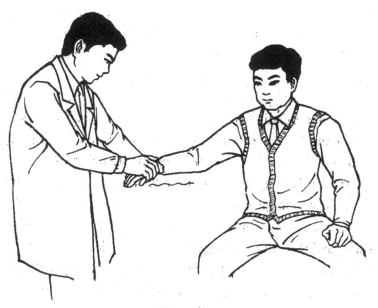

Figure 42

movement along its motor axis and within its physiological limit. Examples of passive movement are flexing and extending forward and backward, flexing laterally left and right, or rotating (See Figure 43).

Essentials. In general, both hands are needed to correctly apply Yao. The force exerted should be steady and slow, and the rotation amplitude should be gradually widened within the physiological limit of the joint. If the rotated joint is in a pathological state such as adhesion, its rotation scope will be markedly narrowed. In this case, the rotating begins with the tolerability of the patient. Larger scope of rotating is then followed gradually; haste is strictly forbidden.

Specifically, one hand holds the upper proximal end of the rotated joint and does not move. The fixed hand protects the joint and ensures that it does not move beyond its physiological limit. It also ascertains that the applied force is transferred to the treated joint, producing curative effect there.

The other hand holds the lower distal end of the rotated joint and rotates the joint. The rotation differs in direction and amplitude based on the structure of the motor axis. Yao is applied to the joints of shoulders, elbows, wrists, finger, knees, toes, and the metacarpophalangeal articulation.

If the rotated joint may be fixed on the bed by the patient's own body weight or by an assistant, the practitioner uses both hands in a single motion to hold the lower distal end of the joint and rotate. In this way, Yao is applied to the joints of the wrist, cervical vertebrae, and lumbar vertebrae.

Application. Applicable to the joints of the cervical vertebrae, lumbar vertebrae, and limbs, this manipulation causes passive movement of joints. Yao lubricates joints, releases adhesions, and improves the function of a joint's movement. Yao is used to treat articular adhesion and stiffness and dysfunction when moving, flexing, or extending.

4.19 Ban (pull)

Explanation. Pull the treated area at both ends of a joint and in two opposite directions.

Essentials. The performance of this manipulation is based on a good command of sports anatomy. You must know the structures of various joints and the number, the motion direction, the motion patterns, the motion amplitude, and the relevant factors of each motor axis. Without this knowledge, there is no hope of determining the correct manipulation position, applying maneuver reasonably—effort-saving, safe, and painless—or producing effective results.

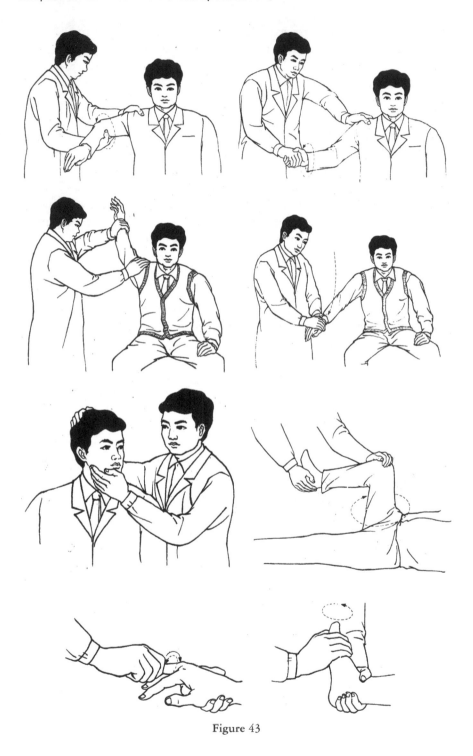

Figure 43

In clinical practice, other manipulations acting on the soft tissues tend to operated around the joints before Ban is used, and Ban is usually used after the spasmodic muscles are relaxed and the contracted ligaments and tendons become normally soft. This has many advantages such as increasing the success rate of Ban manipulation, saving the practitioner's efforts, decreasing the patient's sufferings, and preventing injury due to Ban manipulation.

The following is the introduction to several ways of Ban manipulation.

1. Ban applied to the Neck.

   a. Obliquely pulling the neck. The patient sits upright with his/her head inclined forward about 30. Prop the occiput with one hand and hold the chin with the other. Rotate the head up to its maximum lateral limit (about 45). Repeat in the opposite direction (See Figure 44).

   b. Obliquely pulling for localizing cervical vertebrae. The patient sits upright with the head inclined slightly forward. The practitioner stands behind the patient to perform the manipulation. Use one forearm to hold the patient's head; your elbow is beneath the patient's chin, and your hand is on the patient's occiput. Place the thumb of your other hand on the patient's spinous process of the cervical vertebra; put the other four fingers on the patient's shoulder. The elbow exerts strength first to rotate the head up to the maximum limit (about 45) and then to pull up the cervical vertebra using a rapid rotating/pulling action with small amplitude. Meanwhile, the thumb of the other hand exerts strength in the opposite direction to localize the treated vertebra (See Figure 45).

2. Ban applied to the Chest and Back.

   a. Pulling for chest expansion. This manipulation is applied mainly to the sternocostal joints. The patient sits upright with the fingers of both hands crossed and held on the back of the neck. Stand behind the patient and hold each of the patient's elbows. Support the back of the patient with one of his/her knees. Ask the patient to throw out his/her chest and pull his/her two elbows backwards. While s/he is doing this, help extend the motion by simultaneously pulling the patient's elbows backwards and slightly pushing the back of the patient forward with your knee. The motion should be swift, but in a small range of motion (See Figure 46).

b. Pulling for counter-reduction of the thoracic vertebrae. The patient sits upright with his/her arms raised 180. Standing behind the patient, hold the front of the patient's forearm near the elbow with Hand A and press the affected part of the spine at the back with the thumb of Hand B. Then ask the patient to throw out his/her chest. After the patient does so, pull the patient's arms backwards with Hand A and push the spinous process forwards for its reduction with Hand B. The push with hand B should be reasonably forceful (See Figure 47).

3. Ban Applied to the Waist

a. Obliquely pulling the lumbar vertebrae

i. Obliquely pulling the lumbar vertebrae with patient in a lateral recumbent position. The patient lies in a lateral recumbent position with the lower leg, the hip and knee of the upper leg flexed, the upper arm behind the body, and the lower arm naturally beside the body. Prop the scapulo-anterior of the patient with Hand A and the hip or the anterior superior spine with Hand B. Push the shoulder with Hand A and pull the pelvis with Hand B until the lumbar vertebrae rotate up to the maximum limit. Finally, exert pressure in opposite directions in a small and rapid pressing action (See Figure 48).

ii. Long-handle pattern obliquely pulling the lumbar vertebrae with the patient in the supine position. The patient

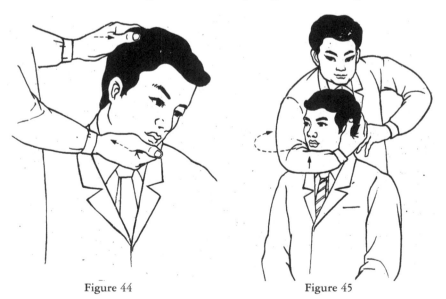

Figure 44   Figure 45

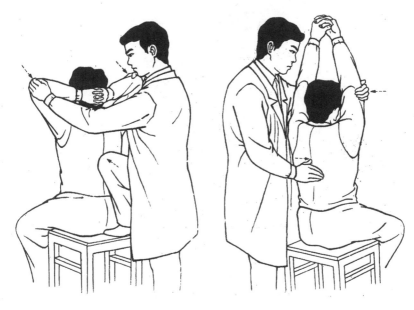

Figure 46   Figure 47

lies supinely with the right arm abducted, the right hip 90 flexed, the right knee flexed, the left arm naturally beside the body, and the left leg extended. Stand on the patient's left and press the scapulo-anterior of the patient with your right hand. Hold the right knee with your left hand (See Figure 49-1), and then press the scapulo-anterior against the bed with your right hand. This action rotates the patient's pelvis to its maximum left limit and his/her thigh parallel to the bed surface. Finally, push/press the leg with

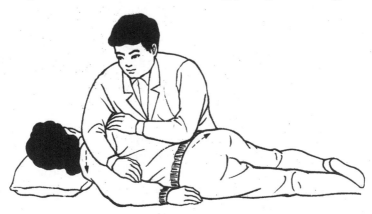

Figure 48

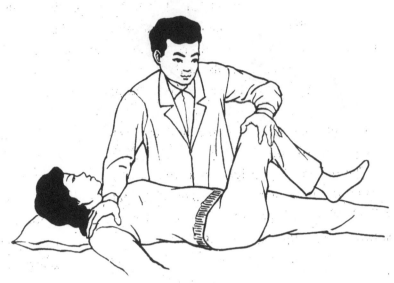

Figure 49-1

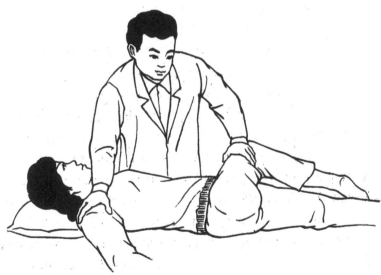

Figure 49-2

your left hand in a downward, rapid and small action (See Figure 49-2). Pulling right, the practitioner stands on the right of the patient, all the other being the same as the above except in the opposite direction.

iii. Obliquely pulling the lumbar vertebrae with a patient in the sitting position. The patient sits upright on a stool with legs apart. Stand beside the patient (either side) and hold the nearest leg of the patient with one hand. With your other hand, hold the other scapulo-anterior of the patient from under the axillary region. Rotate the patient's upper body with force exerted at the same time with both hands so as to pull up the lumbar vertebrae (See Figure 50).

b. Rotating/pulling for reduction of the lumbar vertebrae. The patient sits upright on a stool. For a right rotation, hold the patient's left leg still with your knees and hands. Stand behind the patient on his/her right, and put your left thumb slightly to the right of the patient's spinous process of the treated lumbar vertebra. Ask the patient to bend forward at the waist as far as possible. When in the anteflexed position, stretch the patient's arm to the right by pulling from under his/her right armpit and holding the left side of the patient's neck with the hand.

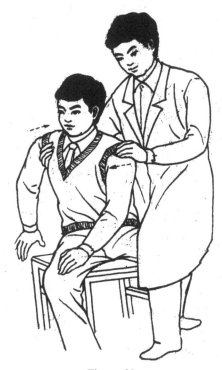

Figure 50

Pull the patient's upper body to the right. Next rotate his/her lumbar vertebrae right by performing a small rapid pulling/rotating action with the right hand (which is still on the spinous process). Follow the maximum rotation of the patient's lumbar vertebrae and at the same time push and press the spinous process left and upward. You should hear a crack or feel that the spinous process is movable (See Figure 51). The process for a left rotation is the same, except that

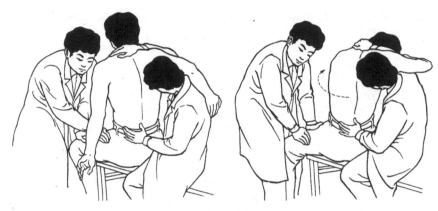

Figure 51

you pull to the left and you may need to reverse your hand positioning.

c. Pulling the lumbar vertebrae backward

    i. Pulling the lumbar vertebrae backward using both legs. The patient lies prone. Support the patient's knees with Hand A and press the affected part of the patient's waist with the palm or palm base of Hand B. Lift the knees slowly until the lumbar vertebrae are extended up to the maximum. With Hand A, rapidly perform a small supporting/lifting action and, at the same time with Hand B, forcefully press downward on the affected vertebra. This pulls up the affected vertebrae (See Figure 52).

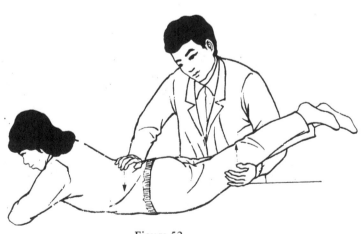

Figure 52

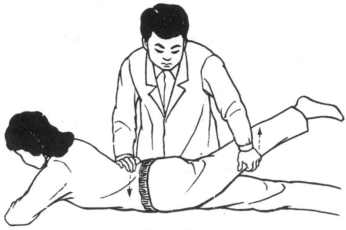

Figure 53

ii. Extending the lumbar vertebrae backward using one leg. The patient lies prone. Stand on the left side of the patient. Hold the patient's right knee with your right hand and press the spinous process of the affected lumbar vertebra with the palm root of the left hand. Slowly raise the patient's right leg and then firmly press the affected vertebra. With your right hand, rapidly lift and pull—a small motion. When the vertebrae are backwards extended up to the maximum, press the palm base of the left hand swiftly downwards. In this way, the lumbar vertebrae slightly overextend so that the affected vertebra can be reduced (See Figure 53). Backward-extending the lumbar vertebrae through lifting the left leg may be performed in the same way.

4. Ban Applied to the Shoulder

a. Pulling the shoulder through abducting. The patient sits upright. Squat on the treated side of the patient. The patient places his/her forearm or elbow on your right shoulder and, using both hands, you press his/her shoulder above the joint (See Figure 54). Rise slowly so as to abduct the patient's shoulder gradually up to the maximum and then stand abruptly so as to have the shoulder abducted to 90. At the same time, press the patient's shoulder downward and hold it firmly with both hands. This manipulation causes stress to reach the shoulder and removes the articular adhesion, restoring motion to the shoulder.

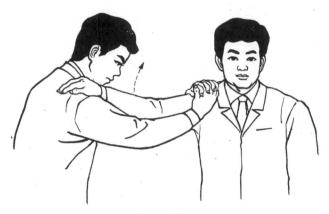

Figure 54

b. Pulling the shoulder via forward-flexing and backward-extending. The patient sits upright. Hold the affected forearm's lower end or the elbow of the patient with Hand A, press the scapulo-posterior with Hand B, and then slowly flex and extend the affected limb forward and backward. When the flexion or extension is done to the maximum, use Hand A to pull up the affected shoulder forward or backward with sudden force. At the same time hold the shoulder still with Hand B by exerting a force against, and in the opposite direction of, the one exerted by Hand A. This strengthens the stress to the shoulder and ensures the curative effects (See Figures 55-1, 55-2 and 56).

In addition, Ban may be also applied to the joints of the elbow, wrist, finger, hip, knee, ankle, and toe. The principle to be followed is as follows: At the same time, apply outward force to the upper and

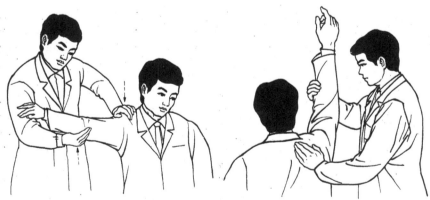

Figure 55-1   Figure 55-2

lower ends of the joint so that the ends are acting against each other. This pulls the joint into an over-extended, over-flexed, over-adducted, or over-abducted position along its motor axis and within its physiological limit.

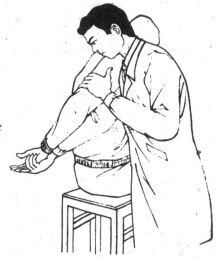

Ban begins steady and slow, but the pulling-up action takes place in the blink of an eye and must be resolute, rapid, and firm. The pulling amplitude is within the normal physiological limit, and the direction of each pull is limited only by one chosen motor axis no matter how many motor axes the pulled joint has. When pulling, the joint will crack. This is a sign that the

Figure 56

pulling stress has reached the required position and the reduction has succeeded. However, clinically, such a sound is not certain to occur to each patient or at each pull. Provided the pulling amplitude is proper, curative effects will result. Therefore, there is no need to keep going until the crack is heard, and it is to widen the pulling range simply to produce this sound. Unnecessary injury of the joint and could ligaments result.

Application. This manipulation is applicable to all the moving joints and every amphiarthrosis, especially to the joints of the neck, lumbar vertebrae, and limbs. It reduces articular disturbance and semiluxation, releases adhesion, lubricates joints, corrects deformity, and restores motion to joints.

4.20 Bashen (pull/extend)

Explanation. Firmly pull and extend both ends of a joint longitudinally in opposite directions so as to prolong the distance and widen the space between the articular surfaces.

Essentials. When Bashen manipulation is performed, the force exerted should be even and lasting, the maneuver should be slow and gentle, and violence is strictly forbidden. As for the direction of the acting force, it should be along the longitudinal axis of the joint. This manipulation must be carefully used to avoid articular deformity and rigidity.

1. Pulling/extending the cervical vertebrae

a. Sitting position. The patient sits upright. Stand behind the patient and prop the occipital bone from below with your thumbs. Support the jaw angles with your palm roots, and press the patient's shoulders with your forearms. Then with force, raise the patient's head with your hands while continuing to firmly press down on the shoulders with your forearms (See Figure 57).

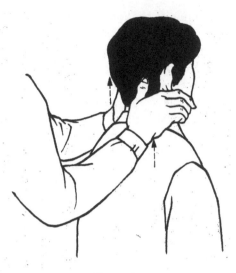

Figure 57

b. Lower sitting position. The patient sits upright on a low stool. Squat halfway and to one side of the patient and prop his/her chin with one elbow. Hold the patient's head tightly with your upper arm and forearm, and support his/her occiput with the other hand (See Figure 58-1). Stretch your upper body so that it is straight, holding the patient's head tightly in your arms. Make sure at this point that the patient relaxes his/her whole body, and then lift the patient's upper body away from the stool by standing. This procedure uses the patient's own body weight to fulfill the traction of his/her cervical vertebrae (See Figure 58-2).

c. Supine position. The patient lies supine without a pillow. Sit in front of the patient's head. Make sure both feet are on the floor and that each of your knees is pressing against the legs of the bed. Lean slightly forward, extend your spine straight, and place your left hand beneath the occiput of the patient and your right hand under the patient's chin. Then holding the patient's head tightly in both hands with your arms stretched straight, exert force with your waist and back to pull the patient's upper body backwards. This causes the patient's body to slide on the bed and, thus, takes advantage of the patient's own body weight to fulfill the traction of the cervical vertebrae (See Figure 59).

2. Pulling/extending the lumbar vertebrae.

a. Prone position. Let an assistant hold both subaxillary regions of the patient in the prone position. If no assistant is avail-

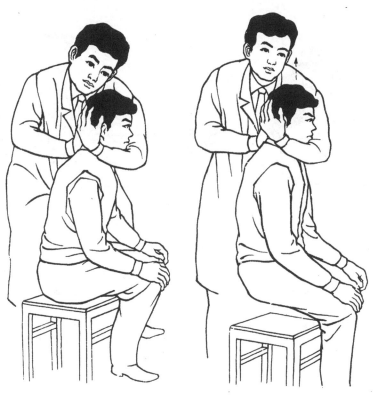

Figure 58-1   Figure 58-2

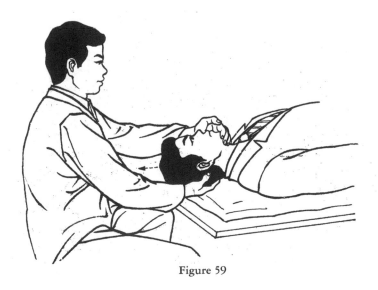

Figure 59

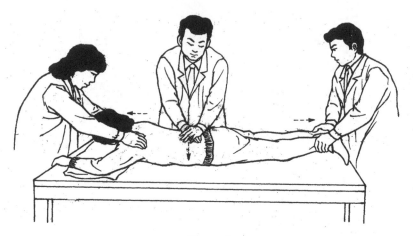

Figure 60

able, ask the patient to hold the bed edge with his/her hands. Grasp the lower ends of the patient's shanks and ask the patient to relax all over or to cough. Just after s/he does, pull/extend the patient's lumbar vertebrae. Work together with the assistant to give forces in the opposite directions (See Figure 60).

b. Carried on the back. The practitioner and the patient stand back against back with elbows linked. Prop the patient's lumbar vertebrae or lumbrosacral portion to be extended with your hips, and ask the patient to cough. Just after the cough,

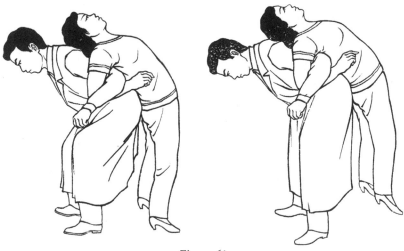

Figure 61

carry the patient on his/her back—feet off the floor—by bending your back, flexing your knees and throwing out your hips. Shake or swing the patient's waist by rhythmically extending your knees and throwing out your hips. The patient's lumbar vertebrae will extend backwards via the weight of his/her own lower body (See Figure 61).

3. Pulling/extending the shoulder. The patient sits on a stool. Hold lower part of the patient's forearm with your hands and ask an assistant to hold the patient's body still. With the

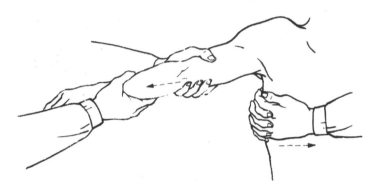

Figure 62

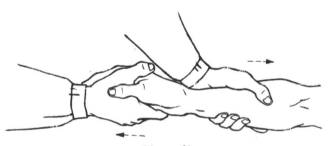

Figure 63

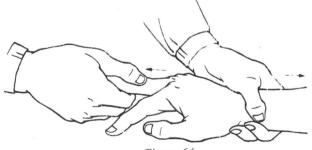

Figure 64

assistant, apply force in opposite directions to slowly pull/extend the shoulder of the patient (See Figure 62). This variation of Bashen can also be performed on elbows, wrists, fingers, hips, knees, ankles, and toes. Use the following principle: Hold the proximal end of the joint with one hand and the distal end with the other. Pull and extend the joint in opposite directions so as to widen its space (See Figures 63 and 64).

Application. Applicable to the cervical vertebrae, lumbar vertebrae and the joints of the four limbs, this manipulation restores and treats injured soft tissues, reduces dislocated joints, widens joint space, remits nerve compression, and releases adhesion. It is one of the main manipulations used to treat cervical spondylopathy, prolapse of lumbar intervertebral disc, torsiversion malposition of tendon ligament, constriction of joint capsule and disturbance, semiluxation, and dislocation of joints.

CHAPTER 5

Basic Training for Performing Manipulations

5.1 Methods for Practicing Manipulations

Tuina professionals must possess the technical ability to perform the maneuvers of every manipulation and the physical endurance and strength to perform the arduous tasks of treatment. To prepare yourself for practicing tuina, you must train your body and mind. To train, perform tuina exercises and, perhaps more importantly, diligently practice the manipulations—especially those with complex makeup and more difficult skills.

While doing tuina exercises, beginners must practice hard, day after day and step by step, strictly according to the basic training methods and steps. Only by doing so, can you acquire superb technique and the ability to perform the manipulations.

There are three stages of basic training, including practicing on a bag filled with rice, practicing on the human body, and practicing through routine performance in treating common diseases. Here is the brief introduction to the training methods and requirements of each stage.

Practice on a Bag Filled with Rice. Except those causing passive movement of joints, all the manipulations need to be practiced on a rice bag. Put rice bag on a table. If practicing Yizhichan Tui, Mo, Rou, or Zhen, sit. Stand if you are practicing Gun. Practice with both the left and right hands.

Practice the manipulations in a fixed position until the technique is satisfactory. Pay great attention to every detail, from the preparatory posture to movement essentials, including the position of the force-giving point, the angle of every moving joint, the swing amplitude, the frequency, body posture while applying the maneuver, breathing, and your state of mind. Ideally, a teacher should point out and correct you while you are practicing. In the beginning, it is most important to perform the maneuver correctly. Only standard maneuvers can lead to the best mechanical state of the manipulations, and, under this state, the necessary force is produced automatically. Once your technique is perfected, you can experiment with the application of greater force if need be.

After you achieve satisfactory consistent performance in the fixed position, begin to practice while moving slowly, to and fro along the longitudinal axis. Practice of these two kinds of techniques lays the foundation for the future performance on the joints and channels of the human body.

Making a rice bag. Stitch a bag 25 cm long and 16 cm wide. Wash enough polished, round grain rice to fill four-fifths of the bag. Put the rice in the bag and sew it closed. Enclose the sewn package in another cloth, and tie (do not sew) the end shut so that you can wash it when dirty. In the beginning, the bag may be tied tight, later on, it may be loosened gradually (See Figure 65).

Practice on the Human Body. The second stage—practice on the human body—is needed to obtain further technical ability and experience in performing manipulations and to lay a good foundation for future clinical application.

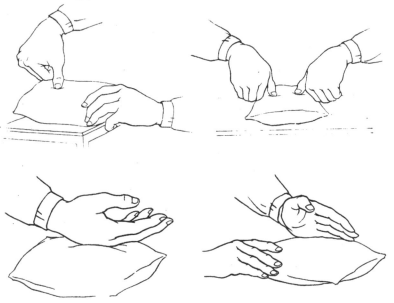

Figure 65

There are two methods for practicing manipulations on the human body. One is to practice various manipulations one by one on each of the channels, collaterals, and points of appropriate parts of the human body. The other is to comprehensively practice and master a few of the manipulations before moving on the another group of manipulations. Either way, repetitive practice and attention to detail (as described above) are essential.

Practice through Routine Performance in Treating Common Diseases. Study during this stage continues to build expertise in the performance of each manipulation. However, it also teaches you how to master the rules for selecting points and working out a prescription through differentiation, as is necessary when tuina is used in clinical practice. Therefore, this is a very necessary training period for the student before s/he really goes to work clinically.

5.2 Exercises

In this section, students will learn about the exercises that are crucial to practicing tuina medicine. The section will highlight benefits, the exercises themselves, and hints for proper execution of the exercises. The benefits of these exercises are evident and proven. Through these exercises, students will:

- Improve the level of his/her health, especially to develop strength, durability, sensibility, and flexibility—essential factors of a successful tuina practitioner.
- Achieve levels of breathing, state of mind, and supplemental nutrients and energy to facilitate the interrelationships within his/her own body. Specifically, the exercises develop the nervous system, endocrine system, internal organs, muscles, joints, and ligaments. This development is needed when s/he is performing any manipulation.
- Ensure the effect and quality of manipulations.
- Enhance the manipulations to raise the curative effects when done in a clinical setting.

Two basic skills are the foundation of basic tuina training exercises: Yijinjing and Shaolinneigong.

5.3. Yijinjing

Yijinjing has 12 forms; five are described below:

Posture of Weituoxianchu (See Figure 66).

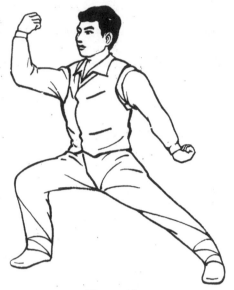

Figure 66

1. Beginning Posture: Stand with the body as upright as possible. Curve the arms with the hands cupped in each other in front of the chest. Breathe evenly and clear the mind. Look natural to purify the spirit.

2. Movements:

   a. Step out with the left foot to set the feet shoulders-width apart. Make sure your feet are parallel to each other and that the soles and toes are fixed on the ground. Keep the legs erect, the popliteal portion slightly relaxed, the head as if supporting an object, the eyes looking straight ahead, the chest harbored, the abdomen restrained, the tongue against the palate, and the mouth slightly open.

   b. Raise the arms laterally to the shoulder level to form a straight line, with the palms facing the ground and the five fingers of each hand closed.

   c. Move both arms forward slowly until the palms meet with the fingertips pointing to the front.

   d. Slowly flex the elbows 90. Keep the wrists, elbows, and shoulders at the same level and the fingertips pointing upward.

   e. Turn the arms and hands slowly inward until the fingertips meet the chest at the level of the point Tiantu (RN 22).

3. Essentials: Do the exercise with rapt attention, but relax the muscles of all parts of the body. Inhale quickly through the nose and exhale slowly through the mouth. When breathing, concentrate the mind on the Dantian and gather *qi* in the lower abdomen—this is called abdomen breathing. In the beginning, do this exercise for three minutes each time. After one to two weeks of practice, increase the time by one to two minutes each week. Do not practice for more than 20 minutes each time.

Note: Doing this exercise persistently helps to develop the strength and durability of the shoulder girdle and the circumflex muscles of the forearm. It improves the flexibility of the wrist so that the ability of the shoulders to suspend can be strengthened along with the durability and flexibility of the forearms to swing.

4. Variations for a patient:

   a. Do the same as (1) in the above.

   b. Move the hands forward until they seem to be holding a ball in front of the chest. Shoulders are 45 abducted; the five fingers of each hand are naturally apart and slightly flexed. Palms are sunken and the five fingertips and the point Laogong of one hand pointing to those of the other one (See Figure 67).

Posture of Zhaixinghuandou (See Figure 68).

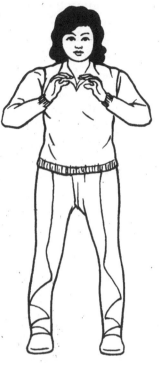

Figure 67

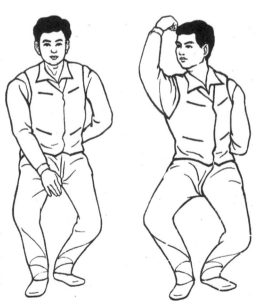

Figure 68

1. Beginning Posture: Stand upright. While doing this exercise, be attentive, breathe in the same way as in Posture of Weituoxianchu to ensure natural breathing.

2. Movements:

   a. Step out a little forward and laterally with the right foot to form a T-shaped stance. The heel of the right foot points to the midpoint of the interior border of the left one with a space of one fist between them. Cup the left hand and rest it against the lumbosacral portion by flexing the elbow backward and, at the same time, hang the right hand anterior to the medial aspect of the right thigh.

   b. Bend the left leg to squat down slowly with the knee about 120-160 flexed. At the same time, lift the heel of the right foot with only the tip of the foot on the ground. Keep the upper body erect; do not lean forward or backward.

   c. Slowly raise the right hand, palm down, from between both legs and along the midline of the abdomen and chest. Keep fingertips together so that they look like a hook.

   d. When the arm reaches the level of the head, adduct the upper arm, rotate the forearm outward, hook the hand, and flex the wrist until the shoulder is 90 protruded, the elbow 90 flexed and the wrist 90-100 bent. Keep the right arm in this posture at the right side of the body.

   e. Turn the hooked fingertips slightly outward as far as possible, while lifting the head slightly right and upward to stare at the center of the palm.

   f. Repeat with the left hand.

   g. Repeat (a) to (f).

3. Essentials: Do not extend the knees past the toes when squatting. Support the weight of the whole body mainly with the back leg, leaving about 30% of the weight for the front leg to bear. Do not raise the hand too high; keep it only one fist high above the head. Pinch the five fingers evenly, and abduct the forearm and laterally-rotated fingertips—and flex the wrist—as far as possible for about ten seconds so that you sense soreness and distension. Do not hold breath when rotating the arm and generating strength.

   Repeat the entire exercise every ten seconds or so during practice time. In the beginning, do this exercise for one to two minutes each time. One week later, add one minute every two weeks until the total practice time is 10-15 minutes.

   Note: This exercise plays a part in strengthening the legs' supporting ability and in developing the strength and endurance of the greater pectoral muscle, the deltoid muscle, the biceps muscle of the arm, the circumlateral muscle of the forearm, and the flexor groups of the wrist. It also elongates the posterior ligament of the wrist and the circum-medial muscle of the forearm to improve their flexibility and anti-pulling ability. This exercise enhances the supporting ability of the shoulder to perform manipulations, the amplitude and durability of the suspended wrist to conduct Yizhichan Tui, the swinging strength and speed of the forearm to perform Gun, and the ability to stand on your feet for long periods of time.

Posture of Daozhuajiuniuwei (See Figure 69).

1. Beginning Posture: Stand upright. Breathing is in the same way as that in the above postures.

2. Movements:

   a. Turn the upper body to the right.

   b. Take a large step forward with the right leg. Flex the right knee 90 to form a forward lunge. Keep the upper body upright and a little sunken.

   c. Clench both hands into fists and face their centers upward. Stretch the arms, one forward and the other backward, with both wrists slightly flexed and both elbows 140-150 flexed. Do not raise the front fist higher than the level of the brows; keep the back fist only as high as the level of the lumbosacral region.

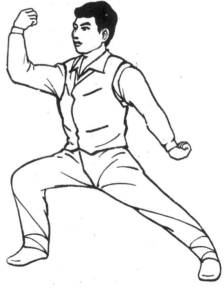

   d. Stare at the center of the front fist. Turn the forearm outward, the backarm inward as if they are twisted like a string. (The strength exerted to do so is called spiral strength and comes from the Dantian.) Harbor the

Figure 69

chest a little, straighten the back, and gather *qi* in the lower abdomen.

   e. Repeat with the left side.

3. Essentials: Positioning of the elbow, knee, and toe is essential to prevent injury and optimize development. If you drew an imaginary line from your elbow down to your toe, the line would be straight, and in no instance would the knee extend beyond the toe or the elbow beyond the knee.

Relax the muscles of the shoulder girdle without lifting the shoulder. Intermittently exert strength with the arm, i.e., twisting an arm up to the time when soreness, distension, and pain are sensed and then hold it for about ten seconds. Start another twisting ten seconds later.

In the first week, do this exercise for three minutes each time. Later on, add one minute each week, until you can perform the exercise for eight to ten minutes per session.

Note: This exercise develops the strength, endurance, and anti-tension ability of the intorter and extortor of the forearm. It helps develop the ability to grasp used in the manipulations Gun, Tui, and Ca.

Posture of Sanpanluodi (See Figure 70).

1. Beginning Posture: Stand upright.

2. Movements:

a. Step out laterally with the left foot to set the feet shoulder-width apart or a little more, with the toes slightly inward.

b. Flex the knees and lower the hips. At the same time, turn the palms upward and raise them slowly to the level of the shoulders from the sides of the body and along the chest.

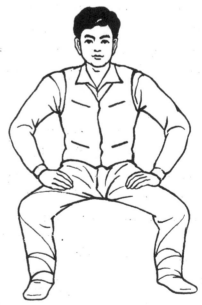

c. Turn the palms upside down and lower them slowly as if pressing something. Keep the fingers naturally relaxed. Put the palms above the knees with the part between the thumb and the index finger towards the body as if holding something. Lean the upper body slightly forward.

d. Turn the upper body upright. Jut the chest out slightly and bow the back.

Figure 70

Relax the muscles of the shoulder girdle, but do not raise the shoulders. Abduct the shoulders about 50; rotate the elbows outward and the forearms inward. Abduct the thumbs, straighten the neck as if there were something on the head. Look straight ahead, keep the mouth slightly open, keep the tongue at rest against the palate, and evenly regulate nasal breathing.

3. Essentials: The extent to which the knees are bent is based on how much a practitioner can do and how much s/he has practiced the exercise. If advanced: the knees are about 160 bent; moderate: about 150-140 bent; conservative: about 100-120 bent. Keep the upper body upright when bending knees, as if sitting on a stool. Do not let the knees protrude over the perpendicular line of the toes.

Do this exercise for one minute each time in the beginning. Later, add one minute each week until total exercise time for this posture is five minutes.

Note: Doing this exercise enhances the strength, endurance, and anti-tension ability of the muscles of the axillae and arms. It strengthens the legs and waist, thus making it easy to stand for long periods, exert strength, and save the energy of the arms while manipulations are being performed.

Posture of Wohupushi (See Figure 71).

1. Beginning Posture: Stand upright.

2. Movements:

   a. Take a large step forward with the left foot and bend the knee at an angle of 90. Stretch the right leg with the toes against the ground, thus forming a left forward lunge.

   b. Extend the arms forward and place the fingertips (not palm) on the ground for support. At the same time, lift the heel of the back foot, raise the head, and look straight ahead.

   c. Relax the front foot and extend the leg backward, put the dorsum of the retired foot on the heel of the back foot, harbor the chest and abdomen a little, straighten the trunk, and hold the head up.

   d. Pull the body backward with the hip protruding backward and the elbows straight.

   e. Bend the elbows slowly, and lower the head and trunk to the front like a prone tiger about to pounce on its prey.

   f. When the head is lowered about 2 *cun* from the ground, slowly stretch the elbows and raise the head and trunk forward and upward.

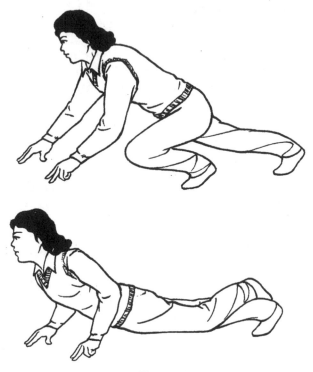

Figure 71

  g. Pull the whole body up, and protrude the hip backward
    again.

  h. Repeat, forming wave-like and repeated movements.

  i. Repeat (a.) to (h.) with the left foot forward.

3. Essentials: Perform this posture slowly, and naturally connect
the raising and the lowering movements. Keep the body
balanced while doing the to-and-fro movements. Move the
upper body slowly forward while exhaling, and integrate the
strength and breathing closely. Never hold your breath.
In the beginning, the fingers and palms may be used for
support. Once you are able to maintain balance, use only the
fingertips, and, finally, use the tips of only three fingers on
each hand: the thumbs, the index fingers, and the middle
fingers.
Note: Doing this exercise can enhance the strength and
endurance of the muscles of the shoulder girdle, the brachial
triceps muscles, and the arms' biceps muscles. It develops
supporting and anti-tension ability of the fingers. Prolonged
practice of it can thicken, strengthen, and toughen the joints,

ligaments, and joint capsules of the fingers. This posture allow you to exert strong and persistent finger and forearm strength, enabling you to protect yourself from being hurt while performing the manipulations Tui, Na, DiAn, An, Ca, and Gun.

5.4 Shaolinneigong

Shaolinneigong consists of many forms. This section explains the basic Shaolinneigong postures and forms.

Standing Posture (See Figure 72).

1. Beginning Posture: Stand upright.

2. Movements:

   a. Set the feet a little more than shoulders-width apart.

   b. Turn the toes of each foot inward.

   c. Plant feet firmly on the ground, lift the head upright, and look straight ahead.

   d. Drop the shoulders, push out the chest, bring the scapulae close to the spinal column, relax the loins, and restrain the lower abdomen.

   e. Harbor the hip slightly, bend the arms, and make sure the thumbs face back and the fingers front.

   f. Breathe naturally.

3. Essentials. To plant the feet, push the whole foot into the ground by rotating the thighs slightly outward while pushing down. Distribute the weight evenly on the toes, heel and arch of your foot. Dig your toes into the ground.

Horse Stance (See Figure 73).

1. Beginning Posture: Stand upright

2. Movements:

   a. Set the feet a little more than shoulders-width apart.

   b. Turn the toes of each foot inward.

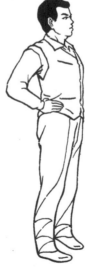
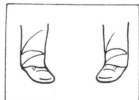

Figure 72

   c. Bend the knees, but not so far that they extend further than your toes.

   d. Squat.

   e. Keep your head upright and look straight ahead.

   f. Push out your chest, straighten the waist, sink the hips but do not let them protrude.

   g. Bend your arms.

    Note: You should look like you are riding a horse.

3. Essentials. There are three levels at which you can squat: high, middle, and low. If your technique and strength are advanced: the knees are about 160 bent; moderate: about 150-140 bent; conservative: about 100-120 bent. Keep the upper body upright when bending knees, as if sitting on a horse. Do not let the knees protrude over the perpendicular line of the toes.

Forward Lunge (See Figure 74).

1. Beginning Posture: Stand upright.

2. Movements:

   a. Set the feet a little more than shoulders-width apart.

   b. Turn the toes of each foot inward and the shank vertical.

   c. Firmly straighten the back leg; the toes are slightly abducted.

   d. Keep the head upright, eyes straight ahead, chest thrown out, waist relaxed, abdomen harbored, hips restrained, and arms bent.

Stretching the Arms and Opening the Palms (See Figure 75).

1. Beginning Posture: Standing posture

2. Movements:

   a. Stand in the beginning posture for several minutes.

   b. Place the palms, face down, on the waist. Close and straighten the four fingers with the thumbs forcefully abducted and perpendicular to them. Dorsi-flex the wrists.

   c. Slowly stretch the arms straight backward and throw out the chest with the scapulae drawn close to the spinal column.

   d. Rotate the forearms forward as far as you can, turning all of the fingers inward. Thumbs and palms should be outward. Do not raise the shoulders, but extend them about 45-30 backward. Straighten the elbows.

   e. Breathe naturally and concentrate the mind to direct *qi* to all parts of the body including the extremities.

3. Essentials: This form is a fundamental training form. It requires straightness of the arms, trunk, and legs and levelness

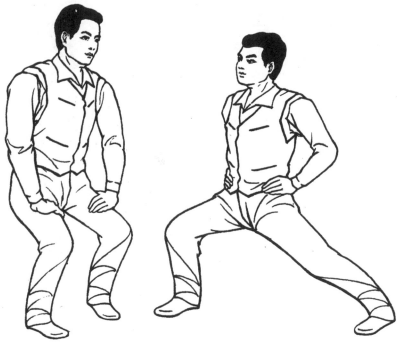

Figure 73   Figure 74

of the head, the shoulders, the palm, and the feet.

Begin practicing for one minute and increase gradually up to ten minutes.

4. Effects:

- Ability to direct *qi* at will
- *Qi* produces essence, which enriches vitality
- Heightened mental state
- *Zang* and *Fu* function well
- *Qi* turns to strength and provides body and the limbs with strength
- Increases strength and endurance of the arms, waist, and legs

Pushing Eight Horses Forward (See Figure 76).

1. Beginning Posture: Standing Posture, Horse Stance, or Forward Lunge. Flex the elbows to 90 with the palms turned upward. Abduct and strengthen the thumbs to make them nearly perpendicular to the other four fingers.

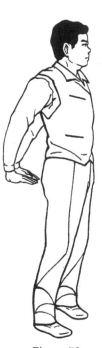

Figure 75

107

2. Movements:

  a. Direct strength to the arms and the fingertips, and push the arms slowly but firmly forward. At the same time, rotate the arms inward until they are at the level of the shoulders with the palms facing each other, the thumbs pointing inward and the elbows fully stretched.

  b. Flex the elbows and withdraw the arms slowly so that the hands return to the hypochondriac region.

  c. Rotate the arms outward and turn the palms upward.

3. Essentials. Practice this exercise in two ways: both arms simultaneously and each arm separately and alternately. Perform each form three to five times. Breathe naturally.

4. Effects:

- Ensures that the legs are strong and can coordinate with the arms

- Increases the ability to of the arms to exert strength

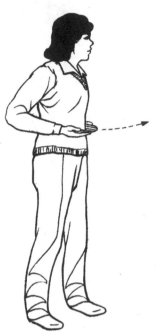

Figure 76

Pulling Nine Oxen Backward (See Figure 77).

1. Beginning Posture: Standing Posture, Horse Stance, or Forward Lunge. Flex the elbows to 90 with the palms turned upward. Abduct and strengthen the thumbs to make them nearly perpendicular to the other four fingers.

2. Movements:

  a. While pushing the arms slowly forward, rotate the forearms slowly inward until the elbows are fully stretched. Turn the palms outward with the dorsums of the hands facing each other and thumbs pointing downward.

  b. Clench the palms into fists and flex the elbows to relax the fists.

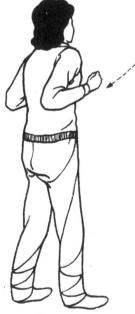

Figure 77

c. Rotate the forearms outward as if pulling a strong ox backward by the tail until the fists reach the costal regions.

d. Extend the fingers with the palms pointing upward (return to the beginning posture).

e. Repeat three to five times, pausing in between each repetition.

An Overlord Holding up a Tripod (See Figure 78).

1. Beginning Posture: Standing Posture, Horse Stance, or Forward Lunge. Flex the elbows to 90 with the palms turned upward. Abduct and strengthen the thumbs to make them nearly perpendicular to the other four fingers.

2. Movements:

a. Firmly and slowly raise the palms, facing upward, as if sustaining a heavy object.

b. As soon as the palms are high above the shoulders, rotate the arms slowly inward until the elbows are fully stretched, with the four fingers of one hand closed and pointing to those of the other, the thumbs abducted and straightened, the palms upward, and the roots of the palms outward.

c. After a pause, rotate the forearms slowly outward until the palms facing the face with the fingertips upward.

d. Firmly lower the palms from in front of the chest to the costal regions.

e. Repeat three to five times, pausing in between each repetition.

Lotus Leaf Swaying in the Wind (See Figure 79).

1. Beginning Posture: Standing Posture, Horse Stance, or Forward Lunge. Flex the elbows to 90 with the palms turned upward. Abduct and strengthen the thumbs to make them nearly perpendicular to the other four fingers.

2. Movements:

a. Firmly and slowly push the palms, face up, upward and forward until the elbows are fully stretched.

b. Cross the palms in front of the chest with the left above the right or vice versa. The distance between them is 1-2 *cun*.

c. Move the arms apart, one leftward and the other rightward. While doing so, keep the palms as if holding up an object.

d. After the shoulders are 90 abducted, move the arms inward until they reach the front.

e. Cross the palms again and draw them to the sides of the waist. Maintain this position for a while.

f. Repeat three to five times.

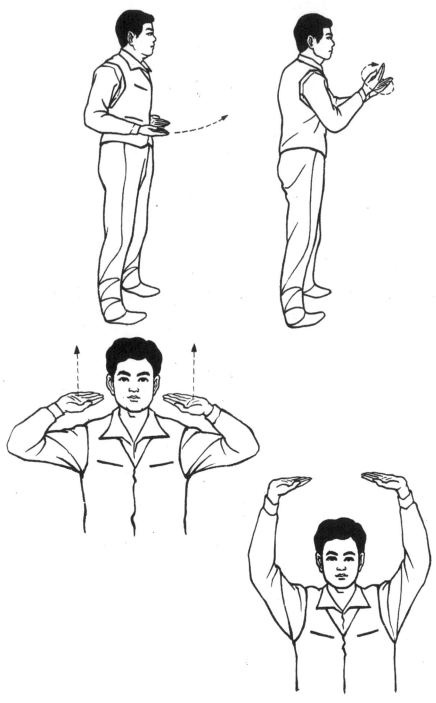

Figure 78

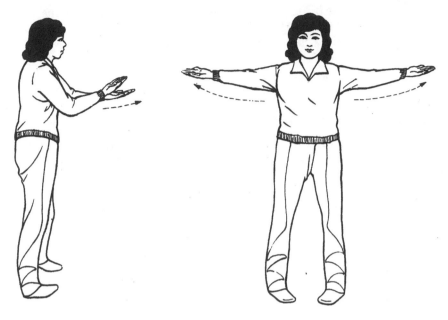

Figure 79

Black Dragon Enters Cave (See Figure 80).

1. Beginning Posture: Wide Forward Lunge with elbows bent and palms stretched at the sides of the waist.

2. Movements:

   a. With palms facing each other, push them slowly forward, turning them inward gradually until they face the ground, the fingertips pointing forward.

   b. Lean the upper body forward. Be sure to stand firm on the bent tips of the toes.

   c. After the elbows are fully stretched, gradually rotate the arms

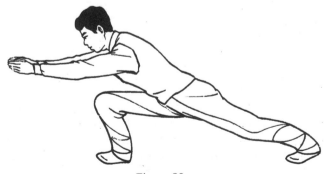

Figure 80

outward until the palms face up. At the same time, flex the elbows (as if something is resisting them) to withdraw the palms to the sides of the costal regions. Maintain this position for a while.

d. Repeat three to five times.

5.5 Attention to Details

- Do the exercises in an orderly way and step-by-step. Reasonably arrange the duration and intensity. Follow the principle "from the simple, the less, and the mild to the complex, the more, and the strong."

- Exercise diligently and perseveringly. It is advisable to practice for 30-60 minutes every day. Doing exercise in "fits and starts" is not helpful or recommended.

- Keep doing the exercise chosen. This is especially important to the beginners, who should not, for example, do Yijinjing or Shaolinneigong today and then practice Baduanjin or Dayangong tomorrow. Tuina students should begin with the basic forms of Yijinjing and Shaolinneigong introduced in this chapter and keep doing them until they have mastered them and become somewhat skilled. Then try some others.

- While training, concentrate your mind. Avoid talking, making jokes, and holding your breath. Do not push yourself unreasoningly. If any abnormality occurs—such as dizziness, chest stuffiness, pain, or irritability—ask a teacher for help in order to prevent deviation or injury. If you do not have a teacher, desist practice. Review the exercise to make sure you are practicing correctly and adjust accordingly. Begin again only when you are feeling well.

- The room in which exercise is done should be quiet, well lit, air-conditioned (or at a comfortable temperature), and well ventilated. Do not expose yourself to cold wind or breezes.

- Wear loose clothes and cloth shoes with soft soles or gym/exercise shoes.

- Morning is the best time for doing exercise. Do not do exercise when the following just occur: Full or empty stomach, strenuous exercise, or tiredness. When finishing or resting, wipe the sweat off with a dry towel and change out of sweaty clothes. Do not fan yourself, take a cold bath immediately, or consume cold food or drink. After the practice is ended, the body may be limbered; to regulate your *qi* and blood, drink warm tea or nutritious beverages to supplement body fluid and nutrients.

- Females should not do exercise when menstruating or pregnant.

CHAPTER 6

Treatment of Common Adult Diseases

6.1 Common Cold

As an exopathic disease common in all four seasons, the common cold manifests mainly as a headache, nasal obstruction, running nose, aversion to wind, and fever. Its course is usually three to seven days.

Etiology and Pathology: It is mainly due to weakness of vital-*qi*, sudden change of weather, and affection of wind-cold or wind-heat. In winter, it is usually due to wind-cold, while in spring, usually due to wind-heat.

1. Cold due to wind-cold: Attack of the superficies of the body by pathogenic cold, obstruction of sweat pores, shut of striae of skin, and dysfunction of the lung-*qi*.

2. Cold due to wind-heat: Heat produced due to retention of wind-cold, heat staying in the superficies of the pulmonary system, and dysfunction of the lung-*qi*.

Clinical Manifestations:

1. Due to wind-cold:

- Chills and fever
- Absence of sweat
- Headache
- Soreness of the limbs
- Nasal obstruction and running nose
- Cough with watery sputum
- Thin and whitish tongue coating
- Floating and tense pulse

2. Due to wind-heat:

- Fever
- Light aversion to wind
- Disturbed sweating
- Pain and distension in the head
- Cough with yellowish and thick sputum
- Sore throat and dry mouth with thirst
- Thin and yellowish tongue coating
- Floating and rapid pulse

Treatment:

1. Therapeutic Method: Expel wind-cold or wind-heat and facilitate the flow of the lung-*qi* to relieve exterior syndrome.
2. Manipulations: Yizhichan Tui, Mo, Na, An, and Rou
3. Point Selection: Fengchi (GB 20), Fengfu (DU 16), Tianzhu (BL 10), Fengmen (BL 12), Feishu (BL 13), Yintang (EX-HN 3), Taiyang (EX-S/HE 5), Touwei (ST 8) and Hegu (LI 4)
4. Operation:
   a. Tui or An and Rou to each of the points Fengchi, Fengfu, Tianzhu, Dazhu (BL 11) and Rengmen five to seven times with the parts around the points manipulated for longer time.
   b. Tui or An and Rou along the line where the points Yintang, Shenting (DU 24), Touwei and Taiyang are located and along the line where the points Yintang, Yuyao (EX-HN 4) and Taiyang are distributed.
   c. Mo from Yintang to Shenting, from Yintang to Taiyang, and along the line where the points Touwei, Shuaigu (GB 8), Naokong (GB 19), and Fengchi are distributed.
   d. Na to Fengchi, the posterior major tendons of the neck, and Jianjing (GB 21).
   e. An and Rou to Fengmen, Jianjing, and Feishu.
   f. Na to Jianjing and Hegu.
5. Supplement
   a. For colds due to wind-cold, Gun is done on Jianjing, Fengmen, and Feishu. Tui is done with the palm over the interscapular region until heat is produced.
   b. For colds due to wind-heat, Tui or An and Rou are done on Fengfu and Dazhui (DU 14); Qia and Rou on Hegu.
   c. For obstruction of the nose, An and Rou on Yingxiang (LI 20).

d. For sore and swollen throat, Qia on Shaoshang (LU 11) and Shangyang (LI 1).

e. For difficulty in coughing up sputum, Rou on Tiantu (RN 22) and Danzhong (RN 17).

6. Treatment Course: Treatment is given once daily for three days.

6.2 Headache

Headache is a subjective symptom. It is common in many acute or chronic diseases.

Tuina is not suitable for the treatment of such intracranial disorders as brain abscess, cerebrovascular disease in its acute period, and intracranial space occupying lesion, brain contusion, and traumatic intracranial hematoma in their acute stages. However, tuina is effective for headaches due to other diseases, especially migraines, muscular contractions, common colds, and hypertension.

Etiology and Pathology:

1. Headache due to exopathy: Improper work and rest and irregular life provide a chance for the six pathogenic factors to invade the body. They go upward along the channels to disturb the lucid *yang*, causing headache.

2. Headache due to internal injury: It may result from the liver impaired by rage, phlegm produced in the spleen, deficient kidney, and insufficient marrow.

Clinical Manifestations:

1. Due to exopathy:

- Headache and stiff neck
- Fever and chills that are worsened by wind
- Nasal obstruction and/or running nose
- Thin and whitish tongue coating or reddened tongue with yellowish coating
- Distending pain and even splitting pain of the head
- Flushed face
- Reddened eyes
- Constipation and/or deep colored urine
- Floating and rapid pulse

2. Due to Hyperactivity of the liver-*yang*:

- Distending head pain
- Vertigo

- Tinnitus
- Vexation and/or irritability
- Insomnia and/or dreamfulness
- Flushed face
- Bitter taste in the mouth
- Reddened tongue with thin and yellowish coating
- Taut, forceful pulse

Treatment:

1. Therapeutic Method: Relieve pain by dispelling wind and removing obstruction in the channels. Headache due to exopathy should be treated by dispelling wind and cold to relieve pain, while headache due to internal injury, by calming the liver to suppress *yang* hyperactivity, promoting blood circulation to remove blood stasis, and dredging the channels.

2. Manipulations: Tui, Na, An, and Mo

3. Point Selection: Yintang (EX-HN 3), Touwei (ST 8), Taiyang (EX-S/HE 5), Yuyao (EX-HN 4), Baijui (DU 20), Fengchi (GB 20), Fengfu (DU 16), Tianzhu (BL 10), Feishu (BL 13), Fengmen (BL 12), and Hegu (LI 4)

4. Operation:

   a. Stand behind the patient in the sitting position. Tui to Fengchi, Fengfu, and Tianzhu for about five minutes.

   b. Let the patient take the sitting posture. Yizhichan Tui from Yintang and Yuyao to Taiyang for five minutes. Then An and Rou to the points Jiaosun (SJ 20) and Baijui for about three minutes.

5. Supplement:

   a. If headache of wind-cold type: Qia and Rou to Dazhui (DU 14), Qichi (LI 11), and Hegu.

   b. In the case of headache of wind-heat type: An and Rou to Feishu and Fengmen.

   c. In the case of headache due to hyperactivity of the liver-*yang*: Ti to Qiaogong, and Qia and Rou to Taichong (LR 3).

6. Treatment Course: Treatment is given once daily for six days.

6.3 Insomnia

Most people do not realize that insomnia includes the following: trouble falling asleep, being easily awakened, fitful or excessive dreaming, and, of course, staying awake all night.

Etiology and Pathology:

1. Thinking too much can impair the heart and spleen. With the heart impaired, *yin*-blood is gradually consumed. With the spleen impaired, food essence cannot be produced, blood cannot be supplemented, and the heart cannot be nourished. Under these conditions, the mind becomes disturbed and causes insomnia.

2. Improper diet hurts the intestines and stomach, leading to retention of food or accumulation of phlegm-heat in the stomach. This will disorder the stomach-*qi* and disturb the mind, causing insomnia. Generally speaking, insomnia is due to *yang* in excess, *yin* in insufficiency, and imbalance of *yin* and *yang*.

Clinical Manifestations:

1. Insomnia due to deficient *qi* and blood in the heart and spleen is marked by:

- Dreamfulness
- Lack of sound sleep
- Palpitation
- Amnesia
- Pale complexion
- Acratia of the limbs
- Emaciation
- Listlessness
- Poor appetite
- Sleeplessness or staying awake all night
- Pale tongue with thin coating
- Thready, weak pulse

2. Insomnia due to deficient *yin* and hyperactivity of fire is marked by:

- Distension of the head
- Deafness and/or tinnitus
- Irritability
- Sleeplessness
- Palpitation
- Restlessness
- Dizziness
- Amnesia

3. Insomnia due to disorder of the stomach-*qi* is marked by:
   - Sleeplessness and/or disturbed sleep
   - Distension and fullness in the stomach and abdomen and/or loss of appetite
   - Hiccups
   - Eructation

4. Insomnia due to weakness in the convalescence is marked by:
   - Weakness of the body
   - Sleeplessness
   - Pale complexion
   - Emaciation
   - Acratia
   - Night sweats or spontaneous sweating
   - Tendency to wake after going to sleep

Treatment:

1. Therapeutic Method: For insomnia of the excess type, sooth the liver to remove heat and regulate the stomach to calm the mind. For insomnia of the deficiency type, strengthen the spleen to replenish *qi* and tranquilize the mind.

2. Manipulations: Na, Mo, An, Rou, and Cuo

3. Point Selection: Fengchi (GB 20), Fengfu (DU 16), Naokong (GB 19), Yintang (EX-HN 3), Jingming (BL 1), Yingxiang (LI 20), Renzhong (DU 26), Chengjiang (RN 24), and Jiaosun (SJ 20)

4. Operation:

   a. Stand behind the patient in the sitting position. Prop his/her forehead with one hand. Open the five fingers of the other hand.

      i. Middle finger on the Du Channel of his/her head.

      ii. Index and ring fingers on the region that the Bladder Channel of Foot-Taiyang goes through.

      iii. Na with five fingers to and fro three to five times from the front hairline to the occipitoposterior region.

      iv. Na to Fengchi and Naokong.

      v. Mo alternately with the bellies of both thumbs to the sternocleidomastoid muscles on both sides of the neck from the above to the below.

      vi. Repeat 10-20 times.

b. Stand directly in front of the patient in the sitting position.

    i. Mo with both thumbs to the area from Yintang to Shenting (DU 24).

    ii. An to Jingming.

    iii. Mo to the area from Cuanzhu (BL 2) to Sizhukong (SJ 23).

    iv. An and Rou with the thumbs to each of all the above points three to five times.

    v. Using the radial sides of the thumbs and alternating from one thumb to the other, Tui rapidly downward from Touwei to Jaosun.

    vi. An and Rou to the points Anmian I (Extra) and Anmian II (Extra).

    vii. Perform each for one to two minutes.

c. Stand at the left or right side of the patient in the sitting position. Prop his/her shoulder with one hand.

    i. Ca to his/her chest repeatedly to and fro and up and down.

    ii. Ca to his/her back.

    iii. Stand behind the patient and Ca to his/her costal regions with both palms until they feel warm.

d. Stand before the patient in the sitting position. Na to Neiguan (PC 6) 50 times and Dianrou to Daling (PC 7) 50 times, both with the right thumb.

5. Treatment course: Treatment is given once daily for 12 days.

6.4 Diarrhea

Diarrhea refers to frequent defecation with thin or even watery stools. In modern medicine, it includes those due to the functional and organic changes of the stomach, intestines, liver, gallbladder, and pancreas, such as acute or chronic enteritis.

Etiology and Pathology: The pathological change of diarrhea takes place in the spleen, stomach, and large and small intestines. Its etiology is both external and internal. Externally, the exopathogens invade the body. Internally, improper diet weakens *zang* and *fu*, causing them to dysfunction. However, the direct cause of diarrhea is as follows: The pathogenic dampness attacks the spleen and weakens it; the weakened spleen malfunctions, and it cannot turn food into essence, and water and dampness are accumulated in the body, causing diarrhea.

Remarkable curative effects are seen when Tuina is used to treat prolonged diarrhea due to weak *zang* and *fu* or decline of the fire from the gate of life.

Clinical Manifestations:

1. Diarrhea due to weakness of the spleen and stomach is marked by:

- Intermittent and repeated loose stools with undigested food
- Frequent defecation, increasing whenever a little greasy food is eaten
- Poor appetite
- Discomfort in the epigastrium occurring after the intake of food
- Sallow complexion
- Listlessness
- Pale tongue with whitish coating
- Slow, weak pulse

2. Diarrhea due to weakness of the kidney-*yang* is marked by:

- Pain around the umbilicus occurring before dawn followed by borborygmus and diarrhea
- Pain relieved after diarrhea
- Cold body and limbs
- Pale tongue with white coating
- Thready pulse

Treatment:

1. Therapeutic Method: Strengthen the spleen, warm the kidney, remove dampness, and relieve diarrhea.

2. Manipulations: Yizhichan Tui, Mo, An, Rou, and Na

3. Point Selection: Zhongwan (RN 12), Qihai (RN 6), Guanyuan (RN 4), Tianshu (ST 25), Zusanli (ST 36), Pishu (BL 20), Weishu (BL 21), and Dachangshu (BL 25)

4. Operation:

   a. The patient is in the supine position.

      i. AnRou along Zhongwan, Shenque (RN 8), and Guanyuan of the Ren Channel to and fro five to six times.

      ii. Mo to the abdomen counterclockwise for about three minutes.

   b. The patient is prone.

      i. Gun for about two minutes along the Bladder channel from top to bottom.

      ii. AnRou to Ganshu (BL 18), Shenshu (BL 23), Pishu, Weishu, and Dachangshu until the sensation of soreness and distension take place.

c. The patient is supine with legs slightly flexed.

   i. AnRou to Zusanli for about two minutes.

   ii. The patient in the prone position. Tui with one thumb from below the tendo calcaneus to Chengshan (BL 57) where you increase the pressure of the maneuver.

   iii. Do the above to and fro seven to eight times.

   iv. Tui in the same way on the other leg.

5. Supplements:

  a. If diarrhea is due to improper diet: Rou to Shangwan (RN 13).

  b. If the hyperactive liver-*qi* attacks the spleen: Rou to Ganshu, Qimen (LR 14), and Zhangmen (LR 13).

  c. If *yang* is deficient in the spleen and kidneys: An to Jingmen (GB 25) and Guanyuan.

6. Treatment Course: Treatment is given once daily for three days.

6.5 Epigastralgia

Epigastralgia is a syndrome of the digestive system whose main symptom is pain in the upper abdomen. It includes gastric ulcer, acute or chronic gastritis, gastrospasm, gastroneurosis, cholecystis, pancreatitis, and cholelithiasis.

Etiology and Pathology:

1. Attack of the stomach by pathogens: Exogenous cold pathogens or eating too much raw and cold food builds coldness in the stomach, causing pain. Eating too much heavy food produces dampness in the interior, causing hot pain or pain due to undigested food.

2. Imbalance between *zang* and *fu*. Epigastralgia may be caused by dysfunction of the liver due to stagnation of its *qi*, original weakness of the spleen and stomach, overstrain, or irregular diet.

Clinical Manifestations:

1. Attack of the stomach by pathogens. Attack by cold pathogens is marked by:

• Sudden pain occurring in the epigastrium that is worsened by cold but relieved by heat

• Local comfort resulted from heat

• Absence of thirst and desire for drink

- Borborygmus followed by watery stools
- Whitish tongue coating
- Tense pulse

Epigastralgia due to retention of food (as a result of pathogen invasion) is marked by:

- Distending pain
- Four eructations
- Acid regurgitation
- Pain relieved after vomiting
- Inability to defecate smoothly
- Thick, greasy tongue coating

2. Imbalance between *zang* and *fu*. Epigastralgia due to insufficient spleen-*yang* is marked by:

- Dull pain in the epigastrium
- Clear and watery vomit
- Comfort resulting from warmth and pressing
- Cold hands and feet
- Loose thin stools
- Light reddish tongue with thin and white coating
- Soft, weak, or deep, thready pulse

Epigastralgia due to stagnation of the liver-*qi* is marked by:
- Belching
- Pain in the hypochondria
- Taut pulse

Tuina is quite effective in treating epigastralgia, especially when the cause is the imbalance between *zang* and *fu*. Tuina should not be used to treat gastroduodenal ulcer in its bleeding stage because it may hematorrhea.

In general, tuina relieves acute stomachache by pressing and kneading forcefully and continuously for about two minutes the pressure pain point on the back or the stomach point on the 2nd metacarpal bone. To cure the root cause and not merely the stomachache, however, you must determine the cause of epigastralgia through careful analysis of symptoms. Specific treatments based on causes are discussed below.

Treatment of Sudden Epigastralgia:
1. Manipulations: An, Rou, Na, and Zhen
2. Point Selection: Ashi (non-fixed point), Ganshu (BL 18), Danshu (BL 19), Pishu (BL 20), Weishu (BL 21), Zusanli (ST

36), Neiguan (PC 6), and the Ashi points around Pishu and Weishu

3. Operation:

a. The patient is in the prone position. Standing at his/her right side, explore with the right thumb along the Bladder Channel of Foot-Taiyang and from the above to the below the pressure pain points around Pishu and Weishu; press them for one minute, and then AnRou either Pishu or Weishu for one to two minutes or until the epigastralgis relieved.

b. The patient is in the supine position. Sitting at his/her right side, use the right thumb and index finger to apply Qia and Na to Neiguan and Zusanli on each side 30-50 times. If the pain does not stop, repeat until it stops.

4. Treatment Course: Treatment is given once daily for three days.

Treatment of Epigastralgia due to Insufficient Spleen-*yang*

1. Point Selection: Shangwan (RN 13), Zhongwan (RN 12), Guanyuan (RN 4), Qihai (RN 6), Geshu (BL 17), Ganshu (BL 18), Pishu (BL 20), Weishu (BL 21), Zusanli (ST 36), and Neiting (SI 44)

2. Manipulations: Yizhichan Tui, An, Zhen, Mo, and Na

3. Operation:

a. The patient is supine. Sit at the right side of the patient.

i. For two to three minutes, apply light, rapid, and gentle Yizhichan Tui repeatedly along Shangwan, Zongwan, Xiawan (RN 10), Qihai, and Guanyuan.

ii. Press Zhongwan with the right middle finger, moving it up and down according to the patient's breath; gradually press harder and maintain this pressure for about one minute. An, Qihai, and Guanyuan each for a half minute, and Mo to Zhongwan for one minute.

iii. Stand up, put both middle fingers on the patient's lumbar portion—one on each side—and thumbs on Tianshu (ST 25) by the umbilicus with one at one side. Work the thumbs and the middle fingers to conduct forceful Na three to five times, and Zhen to Zhongwan with the palm for two minutes.

iv. Na with the right thumb and the middle finger to either Zusanli or Neiting three to five times or until local soreness appears.

b. The patient is prone. Stand at his/her right side.

 i. Apply Yizhichan Tui along the Bladder Channel of Foot-Taiyang on the back; repeat four to five times.

 ii. AnRou with proper pressure to Ganshu, Pishu, Weishu, and Sanjiaoshu (BL 22) for about one to two minutes.

d. Treatment Course: Treatment is given once daily for six days.

For Epigastralgia due to Attack of the Stomach by Hyperactive liver-*qi*:

1. Point Selection: Qimen (LR 14), Zhangmen (LR 13), Jiquan (HT 1), and Jianjing (GB 21)

2. Manipulations: An, Mo, Na, and Mo

3. Operation:

 a. The patient is supine. Sit at the right side of the patient.

 i. Mo for two to three minutes along the liver region.

 ii. An to either Qimen or Zhangmen for one minute.

 b. The patient sits upright with his/her hand holding his/her own hands.

 i. Mo 40-50 times with both palms from the armpit to the anterior superior iliac spine.

 ii. Na to Jiquan three to five times.

 iii. Na to Jianjing three to five times.

4. Treatment Course: Treatment is given once daily for six days.

6.6 Hemiplegia due to Apoplexy

Tuina is effective in treating hemiplegia to a certain extent, for it can promote the recovery of the body's function. If early treatment with Tuina is given, better curative effects will result. Hemiplegia is usually due to hypertensive apoplexy.

Etiology and Pathology: Invasion of wind-phlegm into the channels and collaterals obstructs the blood vessels and stagnates *qi* and blood. When this happens, the channels and collaterals are blocked, *qi* fails to flow, blood fails to nourish *zang* and *fu*, and hemiplegia results. Damage of the cerebral bone and meninges due to direct or indirect trauma also stagnates blood and obstructs the channels and collaterals causing hemiplegia.

Clinical Manifestations:

• Paralysis of the arm and leg of one side of the body

• Distortion of the eyes and mouth

- Stiff tongue
- Dysphasia

Notes: In the beginning, the affected limbs become soft and weak with impaired perception and motor function. Then the limbs grow stiff and spasmodic. Over a long period of time, the disease will change or distort the limbs.

Treatment:

1. Therapeutic Method: Promote blood circulation to remove blood stasis and activate the *qi* flow to relax the muscles and tendons. It is advisable to give treatment two weeks after the onset.

2. Point Selection: Fengchi (GB 20), Jianjing (GB 21), Jianyu (LI 15), Quchi (LI 11), Shousanli (LI 10), Hegu (LI 4), Zusanli (ST 36), Xinshu (BL 15), Ganshu (BL 18), Shenshu (BL 23), and Weizhong (BL 40)

3. Manipulations: Yizhichan Tui, Gun, An, DiAn, Nian, and Yao

4. Operation:

   a. The patient is prone.

      i. Gun along the Bladder Channel of Foot-Taiyang at both sides of the spinal column from the above to the below for two minutes.

      ii. An mainly on Xinshu, Ganshu, Pishu (BL 20), Feishu (BL 13), and Shenshu.

      iii. Gun on the hip portion, the posterior aspect of the thigh, popliteal fossa and the posterior aspect of the shank.

      iv. AnRou mainly on Chengfu (BL 36), Yinmen (BL 37), Weizhong, Chengshan (BL 57), Kunlun (BL 60), and Taixi (KI 3).

      v. Flex and then rotate the patient's hip and knee inward or outward many times.

   b. Stand at one side of the patient in the supine position.

      i. Gun on the interior aspect of the affected arm from above to below along the forearm and especially around the shoulder, elbow, and wrist for three to five minutes. While doing so, abduct the shoulder, flex the elbow, and flex, extend, rotate the wrist.

      ii. Nian with the thumb and the index finger to each finger of the affected arm, especially to the thumb.

5. Treatment course: Treatment is given every two days, 15 treatments over 30 days.

6.7 Flaccidity Syndrome

Flaccidity syndrome is marked by:
- Loosened and weak muscles and tendons which have been unable to move voluntarily for a prolonged period of time—often in the legs
- Myophagism
- Loss of control of the hands and feet
- Paralysis such as:
- Multiple neuritis
- Myelitis
- Progressive myatrophy
- Myasthenia gravis
- Periodic paralysis
- Myodystrophia
- Hysterical paralysis and sequalae of infection of the central nervous system

Etiology and Pathology:

1. Affection of wind-heat: Invasion of exogenous wind-heat into the lung impairs the body fluid in it and fails to moisten muscles and tendons.
2. Retention of damp-heat: Retention of damp-heat in the interior exhausts the body fluid and fails to lubricate joints.
3. Deficient *yin* of the liver and kidneys: General debility and intemperance in sexual life consume the essence of the liver and kidney and fails to nourish muscles and tendons.

Clinical Manifestations:

1. Due to lung-heat: Impaired production of body fluids usually appears after epidemic febrile diseases and manifests as:
- Sudden loss of control of the weak limbs
- Vexation
- Thirst
- Constipation
- Deep colored urine
- Reddened tongue with yellow coating
- Thready and rapid pulse
2. Due to deficient *yin* of the liver and kidney: Impaired production of body fluids usually appears during a prolonged disease and is marked by:

- Soft limbs or loss of control of the leg
- Emaciated muscles
- Soreness and weakness of the loins and knees
- Vertigo
- Thready and rapid pulse

3. Due to spleen and stomach weakness: Impaired production of body fluids appears after severe or prolonged diseases and is marked by:

- Gradual loss of control of the weak legs
- Lassitude
- Acratia
- Poor appetite
- Loose stools
- Pale complexion
- Pale tongue with thin and whitish coating
- Soft and thready pulse

4. Due to retention of damp-heat: Impairment of the production of body fluids is marked by:

- Paralysis
- Slight swelling and numbness of the legs
- Fullness in the chest and epigastrium
- Sallow body and face
- Deep colored urine
- Difficulty and hot pain during urination
- Reddened tongue with yellow and greasy coating
- Soft and rapid pulse

Treatment:

1. Therapeutic Method: Nourish *yin* to strengthen the stomach and regulate liver, spleen, and kidneys.
2. Point Selection: Jianyu (LI 15), Quchi (LI 11), Hegu (LI 4), Yangxi (LI 5), Biguan (ST 31), Futu (ST 32), Liangqiu (ST 34), Zusanli (ST 36), and Jiexi (ST 41)
3. Manipulations: Gun, An, Rou, and DiAn
4. Operation:
   a. The patient is supine. Sit at one side and hold the affected limb with the left hand.
      i. Gun with the right hand for three to four minutes along

Jianyu, Quchi, Hegu, and Yangxi of the Large Intestine Channel of Hand-Yangming.

    ii. AnRou each of the points selected for one minute.

    iii. DiAn each point for 30 seconds.

    iv. Flex and extend the arm.

  b. Take the same position as above.

    i. Gun to the leg for three to four minutes in the direction of the Stomach Channel in the leg.

    ii. AnRou each of the points Biguan, Liangqiu, Zusanli and Jiexi for about one to two minutes.

    iii. Qia to the nail root of each toe and the interphalangeal joints of the hand.

    iv. Nian to each of the fingers from top to bottom.

    v. Repeat all the above maneuvers seven to eight times.

5. Supplements:

  a. Qia and Rou to Quchi, Hegu, and Sanjinjiao (SP 6) for impaired function due to lung-heat.

  b. Rou to Pishu, Weishu, Shousanli, and Zusanli for impaired function due to spleen and stomach weakness.

  c. Rou to Ganshu, Shenshu, Xuanzhong (GB 39), and Yanglingquan (GB 34) for impaired function due to deficient liver and kidney *yin*.

  d. Rou to Pishu and Fenglong (ST 40) for retention of damp-heat.

6. Treatment Course: Treatment is given every two days, 15 treatments over 30 days.

6.8 Arthralgia syndrome

Arthralgia syndrome is due to stagnation of *qi* and blood by pathogens.

Etiology and Pathology:

Pathogenic wind, cold, and dampness invade the channels and collaterals in the superficies of the body. These pathogens obstruct channels and collaterals and stagnate *qi* and blood, resulting in pain, soreness, numbness and heavy sensation in the limbs, joints, muscles, and tendons.

Clinical Manifestations:

1. Arthralgia due to wind-cold-dampness:

  • Pain in the joints of the four limbs or to the lumbodorsal region and that is aggravated by movement

- No local redness and swelling or aversion to wind
- Migrating pain or pain that worsens with cold but is relieved by heat
- Heavy sensation in the limbs
- White and greasy tongue coating
- Tense or taut pulse

2. Arthralgia due to wind-damp-heat:

- Redness
- Swelling and pain of the joints that are relieved by cold but aggravated by pressure
- Limited joint movement
- Fever
- Thirst and dry throat
- Yellow and dry tongue coating
- Slippery and rapid pulse

Treatment:

1. Therapeutic method: Treat arthralgia due to wind-cold-dampness by dispelling wind, cold, and dampness. Treat arthralgia due to wind-damp-heat by dredging the channels and collaterals.

2. Point Selection: Jianjing (GB 21), Quchi (LI 11), Hegu (LI 4), Huantiao (GB 30), Yinlingquan (SP 9), Yanglingquan (GB 34), Heding (EX-LE 2), Kunlun (BL 60), Fengchi (GB 20), Dazhui (DU 14), Feishu (BL 13), Shenshu (BL 23), Dachangshu (BL 25), and Xiaochangshu (BL 27)

3. Manipulations: Gun, DiAn, An, Rou, and Ca

4. Operation:

   a. First apply manipulations selected according to the affected joints. Then apply Nian and Bashen. Functional movement is suitable for the limited joints.

   b. Yizhichan Tui or Gun gently on the affected joints for three to five minutes. Then the operation gradually shifts to the affected joints.

   c. An Dazhui 20-30 times and Na either Quchi or Hegu five times.

5. Supplement:

   a. For arthralgia due to heat. Qia and Rou to Dazhui, Quchi, and Hegu.

     b. For migrating arthralgia: AnRou to Baihui (DU 20), Fengfu (DU 16), and Fengchi.

  6. Treatment Course: Treatment is given once daily for 12 days.

6.9 Hypertension

Hypertension is marked mainly by dizziness and distension in the head and is, of course, measured by a blood pressure that exceeds 140/90.

Etiology and Pathology:

Causes of hypertension include:

1. Prolonged nervousness, vexation, or anxiety leads to stagnation of liver-*qi*; prolonged stagnation of the liver-*qi* results in fire, and fire consumes liver-*yin*. In this case, consumed *yin* cannot restrict *yang*, and, thus, liver-*yang* becomes overactive.

2. Insufficient kidney-*yin* due to senility causes liver malnourishment, causing hyperactivity of the liver-*yang*.

3. Consuming too much greasy food or alcohol produces phlegm-dampness in the interior; prolonged accumulation of phlegm-dampness forms heat, and heat burns body fluid and turns it into phlegm. Phlegm, in turn, blocks the channels and collaterals.

Clinical Manifestations:

Generally:

- Dizziness and distending pain in the head
- Tinnitus
- Blurred vision
- Irritability
- Choking sensation in the chest
- Palpitation
- Flushed face
- Reddened eyes
- Numbness of the fingers
- Dry mouth and throat
- Constipation
- Deep colored urine
- Reddened tongue with yellow coating
- Taut and rapid pulse

  1. Hypertension due to retention of phlegm-dampness:

- Headache
- Dizziness
- Heavy sensation in the head
- Full sensation in the chest and epigastrium
- Tendency to vomit, even vomiting phlegm and saliva
- White and greasy tongue
- Taut and slippery pulse

2. Hypertension due to hyperactivity of the liver-*yang*:
- Dizziness
- Headache
- Flushed face
- Reddened eyes
- Bitter taste in the mouth
- Irritability with an inclination to be angry

3. Hypertension due to deficient *yin* and *yang*:
- Vertigo
- Headache
- Tinnitus
- Palpitation
- Dyspnea due to movement
- Soreness and weakness of the loins and knees
- Insomnia and/or dreamfulness
- Frequent urination at night
- Pale or reddish tongue with whitish coating
- Taut and thready pulse

Treatment:
1. Therapeutic Method: Calm the liver and remove phlegm.
2. Point Selection: Baihui (DU 20), Sishencong (EX-HN 1), Fengchi (GB 20), Jianjing (GB 21), and Qiaogong
3. Manipulations: An, Rou, Qia, and Na
4. Operation:
   a. The patient is sitting, and should remain so for about five to six minutes before you start.
      i. AnRou to Baihui.
      ii. Mo his/her head with the palm.
      iii. An forcefully to Sishengcong.

    iv. Na to Fengchi with the thumb and index finger.

    v. Na to Jianjing several times.

  b. The patient is prone. Ca with the hypothenar dozens of times from top to bottom along the Bladder Channel in the back.

  c. The patient is sitting. Stand to one side and hold the patient's head with one hand.

    i. Tui downward with the index and middle fingers over Xiaogong with the trail connecting Yifeng (SJ 17) posterior to the ear and Quepen (ST 12). Repeat for about five minutes.

    ii. Repeat (i.) on the other side.

5. Supplements:

  a. Qia and Rou to Xingjian (LR 2), Shenmen (HT 7), and Shaohai (HT 3) for severe headache and dizziness.

  b. Qia and Rou to Zusanli (ST 36) and Sanyingjiao (SP 6) for insomnia, lassitude, and sallow complexion.

6. Treatment Course: Treatment is given once daily for 15 days.

Note: When Tui is applied over Qiaogong, performance on both sides at the same time is strictly forbidden.

6.10 Hiccups

Hiccups are due to *qi* rising from below the diaphragm. They manifest as sudden, sharp, and frequent sounds in the throat. The onset is intermittent and uncontrollable.

Etiology and Pathology:

Causes of hiccups are:

1. Improper diet leads to accumulation of food in the middle-*jiao*, which impairs the spleen and stomach and causes stomach-*qi* to ascend adversely. The adverse ascension of stomach-*qi* is responsible for hiccup.

2. Vexation and anger hurt the liver. The hurt liver malfunctions and disrupts *qi* flow. In this case, phlegm is produced and the spleen is attacked. Ascending of the phlegm along with the adverse flowing of liver-*qi* is responsible for hiccup.

3. Debility due to prolonged disease consumes stomach-*yin*. Insufficient stomach-*yin* makes the stomach unable to be nourished causing hiccups.

Clinical Manifestations:

1. Hiccups due to deficiency syndrome:

  • Hiccups with low sound

- Pale complexion
- Poor appetite
- Sleepiness
- Shortness of breath
- Palpitation
- Weakened voice
- Pale tongue with white coating
- Deep, thready, and weak pulse

2. Hiccups due to excess syndrome:
   - Continual, loud, and forceful hiccups
   - Distending pain in the chest and hypochondria
   - Foul breath
   - Restlessness
   - Thirst
   - Constipation
   - Brown urine
   - Yellow tongue coating
   - Slippery and rapid pulse

3. Hiccups due to cold syndrome:
   - Weak, quiet hiccups accompanied by dyspnea and relieved by heat
   - Poor appetite
   - Absence of thirst
   - Cold limbs worsened by cold
   - White and moist tongue
   - Slow pulse

4. Hiccups due to heat syndrome:
   - Loud hiccups
   - Halitosis
   - Restlessness
   - Preference for cold drinks
   - Dry mouth and tongue
   - Flushed face
   - Reddened eyes
   - Reddish tongue with yellow coating
   - Rapid pulse

Treatment:

1. Therapeutic Method: Regulate the stomach to make the adverse *qi* flow descend.

2. Point Selection: Cuanzhu (BL 2), Yuyao (EX-HN 4), Quepen (ST 12), Danzhong (RN 17), Zhongwan (RN 12), Geshu (BL 17), Weishu (BL 21), Dachangshu (BL 25), Zhongkui (EX-UE 4), Zusanli (ST 36), Fenglong (ST 40), and Neiguan (PC 6)

3. Manipulations: Qia, An, Rou, Mo, and Yizhichan Tui

4. Operation:

   a. The patient is supine. Sit at one side of the patient.

      i. Qia with the nails of both thumbs to Cuanzhu (both sides) and Yuyao for one minute each.

      ii. If the hiccups stop, conduct light, rapid, and gentle Yizhichan Tui on Danzhong and Zhongwan for 1-2 minutes each. Mo clockwise on Zhongwan for three to five minutes.

      iii. Na to Zusanli and Fenglong three to five times each.

   b. The patient is prone.

      i. Yizhichan Tui with the right thumb for three to four minutes each.

      ii. DiAn forcefully with the middle finger to Geshu and Weishu three to four times each.

      iii. AnRou to Dachangshu 20-40 times.

   c. The patient is sitting. Hold his/her left hand with the left hand to flex his/her middle finger.

      i. Qia to Zhongkui on the radius aspect of the second interphalangeal joint of the flexed middle finger for one minute. Use the thumbnail.

      ii. Na to Quepen three to five times.

      iii. Na to Neiguan three to five times.

5. Treatment Course: Treatment is given one time daily for three days.

6.11 Uroschesis

Uroschesis refers to difficulty in urination or even retention of urine.

Etiology and Pathology:

The onset of this disease is mainly related to dysfunction of tri-*jiao-qi* and of the lungs, spleen, and kidneys. Causes include:

- Abundant lung-heat
- Damp-heat in the bladder
- Insufficient kidney-*yang*
- *Qi*-deficient lungs and kidneys
- Traumatic injury
- Accumulation of blood stasis

Clinical Manifestations:

1. Uroschesis due to damp-heat in the bladder:

- Difficulty urinating
- Dribbling urine
- Scanty, deep colored urine
- Burning sensation when urinating
- Retention of urine
- Difficult defecation
- Reddened tongue with yellowish, greasy coating
- Soft and rapid pulse

2. Uroschesis due to abundant lung-heat:

- Difficulty urinating
- Dribbling urine
- Dry mouth and throat
- Restlessness
- Thirst
- Shortness of breath
- Reddened tongue with yellowish coating
- Rapid pulse

3. Uroschesis due to deficient kidney-*yang*:

- Dribbling urine
- Difficulty urinating and defecating
- Cold lower abdomen
- Soreness and weakness of the loins and knees
- Pale complexion
- Pale, enlarged, and tender tongue with whitish coating
- Deep and thready pulse

Treatment:

1. Therapeutic Method: Promote the functional activity of *qi* to reduce difficulty in urination.

2. Manipulations: An, Rou, and Tui

3. Point Selection: Liniao, Dantian, Sanyinjiao (SP 6), and Jimen (SP 11)

4. Operation:

   a. The patient is supine. Calm his/her mind and stand at the side of the patient.

      i. An with the middle finger on Liniao at the midpoint of the line connecting the umbilicus and Zhongji (RN 3). Gradually add pressure becoming as forceful as the patient can endure. If mild or moderate pressure results in urination, heavy pressure is not needed. After the urination is stopped, take away the middle finger slowly. If urination does not occur, An to Dantian for three to five minutes.

   b. The patient is supine with the legs stretched straight and a little abducted. Powder the inner legs with a thin layer of talc powder.

      i. Tui 1000 times from the interior aspect of the knee via Jimen to the groin.

      ii. Ten minutes after completing (i.), ask the patient to urinate.

   c. Na to Sanyinjiao three to five times and Yao each of the ankles five to ten times.

5. Treatment Course: Treatment is given one time daily for three days.

6.12 Constipation

Constipation refers to difficulty in defecation and prolonged interval between the times one defecates. The large intestine retains feces too long, and this dries the feces, making it difficult to discharge.

Etiology and Pathology:

The causes of constipation are:

- General excessive *yang* and addiction to pungent and greasy food lead to accumulation of heat in the stomach and intestines

- Heat that lingers after febrile disease consumes body fluid

- Deficient *qi* and blood due to senile infirmity is responsible for dysfunction of the large intestine and for scanty body fluid.

Clinical Manifestations:

1. Constipation due to excess *yang*:

   • Dry feces
   • Scanty and brown urine
   • Flushed face
   • Fever or distending abdomen
   • Dry mouth
   • Restlessness or frequent belching
   • Fullness in the chest and hypochondria
   • Poor appetite
   • Reddened tongue with a yellow, dry coating
   • Slippery and rapid pulse

2. Constipation due to deficient *qi*:

   • Difficult defecation
   • Slightly dry feces
   • Forced defecation followed by tiredness and even sweating and shortness of breath
   • Pale complexion
   • Lassitude
   • Pale tongue with thin coating
   • Weak pulse or clear and abundant urine
   • Cold limbs or cold pain of the loins and knees or abdomen

Treatment:

1. Therapeutic Method:

   a. Due to excess *yang*: Clear away heat to moisten the intestines. Promote *qi* flow to remove stagnation.

   b. Replenish *qi* to nourish blood and relieve constipation through warming.

2. Manipulations: Mo, An, Rou, and Ca

3. Point Selection: Tianshu (ST 25), Zhongwan (RN 12), Shenque (RN 8), Qihai (RN 6), Pishu (BL 20), Weishu (BL 21), Ganshu (BL 18), Dachangshu (BL 25), Baliao (BL 31-34), Changqiang (DU 1), Zhigou (SJ 6), and Chengshan (BL 57)

4. Operation:

   a. The patient is supine. Stand at one side of him/her.

      i. Mo clockwise over the abdomen with the palm for about five minutes.

      ii. AnRou on Tianshu, Zhongwan, Shenque, and Qihai for about two minutes.

   b. The patient is prone.

      i. Ca with the hypothenar from the patient's waist to the coccyx for about two minutes.

      ii. AnRou to Pishu, Shenshu, and Dachangshu several times each.

   c. The patient is sitting. Qia and Rou to Zhigou and Shangjuxu (ST 37) for about three minutes.

5. Treatment Course: Treatment is given once daily for six days.

6.13 Angina Pectoris

Angina pectoris manifests primarily as paroxysmal and continuous pain in the precordial region behind the sternum. It is due to obstruction of *qi* in the chest.

Etiology and Pathology:

The onset of this disease is caused by or related to:

- Insufficient kidney-*qi* due to senile infirmity
- Impairment of the spleen and stomach due to a rich, fatty diet
- Stagnation of *qi* and blood due to accumulation of liver-*qi* resulting from mental disorder

Clinical Manifestations:

1. Angina Pectoris due to stagnation of *qi* and blood/obstruction of the heart collaterals:

- Paroxysmal stabbing pain in the precordial region
- Choking and oppressed sensation in the chest
- Dyspnea
- Dark tongue with petechiae on the margins and tip
- Deep, uneven, or knotted pulse

2. Angina Pectoris due to deficient *yang-qi* in the upper-*jiao*:

- Choking and oppressed sensation in the chest
- Paroxysmal pain in the heart
- Palpitation
- Shortness of breath
- Dyspnea
- Pale complexion
- Lassitude

- Acratia
- Chills
- Cold limbs or spontaneous sweating
- Disturbed sleep
- Poor appetite
- Clear and abundant urine and loose stools
- Pale, enlarged, and tender tongue with whitish, moist, or greasy coating
- Deep, slow or knotted, and intermittent pulse

3. Angina Pectoris due to deficient *yin* and *yang*:
- Choking sensation in the chest
- Pain of the heart
- Waking up in the night due to dyspnea
- Palpitation
- Shortness of breath
- Dizziness
- Tinnitus
- Poor appetite
- Weakness of the limbs
- Soreness of the loins
- Cold limbs
- Fever in the palms
- Frequent urination
- Purple, dark tongue with whitish and dry coating
- Thready, weak or knotted, and intermittent pulse

Treatment:

1. Therapeutic Method: Promote blood circulation to remove blood stasis and activate the *qi* flow to dredge the collaterals.

2. Manipulations: Mo, An, Rou, and DiAn

3. Point Selection: Yunmen (LU 2), Zhongfu (LU 1), Rugen (ST 18), Qimen (LR 14), Zhangmen (LR 13), Jiquan (HT 1), Jueyinshu (BL 14), Feishu (BL 13), Xinshu (BL 15), Ganshu (BL 18), Shenshu (BL 23), Mingmen (DU 4), Neiguan (PC 6), Daling (PC 7), and Yongquan (KI 1)

4. Operation
   a. Sit to the left of the patient who is supine.
       i. Slow, gentle, and steady Mo with the right palm from top

to bottom on Zhongfu, Yunmen, Qimen, and Zhangmen for five minutes.

    ii. Na gently to Jiquan three to five times.

b. Sit to the left of the patient who is supine. Hold his/her left hand with the left hand.

    i. AnRou either Neiguan or Daling 50 times with the thumb.

    ii. Repeat on the other side.

c. The patient is sitting or lateral. Stand to one side.

    i. Yizhichan Tui on Feishu, Jueyinshu, Xinshu, Ganshu, and Shenshu 100 times each.

5. Supplement:

a. Due to stagnation of phlegm:

    i. Rou to Zusanli (ST 36) 300 times.

    ii. Rou to either Pishu or Wishu 300 times.

b. Due to deficient *yin* and *yang*:

    i. Mo to either Shenshu or Mingmen 300 times.

    ii. Cuo to Yongquan (KI 1) 300 times.

    iii. Mo with the palm the left upper part of the back where Jueyinshu (BL 14) and Xinshu are located for five minutes.

    iv. An gently to either Shenshu or Mingmen three to five times.

6. Treatment Course: Treatment is given once daily for 15 days.

Note: Gentle manipulations and a non-prone position are suggested to avoid worsening choking and palpitation.

6.14 Colicky Pain of the Gallbladder

Colicky pain of the gallbladder is a common symptom of digestive system diseases, such as acute cholecystitis, cholelithiasis, and biliary ascariasis.

Etiology and Pathology:

The gallbladder is exteriorly-interiorly related to the liver and has the same function as the liver in dredging; its *qi* normally flows downward. Stagnation of *qi* of the liver and gallbladder are due to:

• Anxiety and anger

• Disorder of gallbladder-*qi* due to accumulation of damp-heat in the middle-*jiao*

• Dysfunction of the spleen and stomach caused by improper diet

Clinical Manifestations:

Colicky pain due to *qi* stagnation:

- Distending, colicky, or paroxysmal wandering pain in the hypochondriac regions
- Bitter taste
- Dry throat
- Loss of appetite
- Slightly reddish tongue tip
- Thin, whitish, or slightly yellow tongue coating
- Taut and tense pulse

2. Colicky pain due to damp heat:

- Continuous distending pain accompanied by paroxysmal pain sometimes in the hypochondriac regions
- Bitter taste
- Dizziness
- Alternate attack of chills and fever
- Sallow eyes and body
- Yellow, turbid, or brown urine
- Difficult urination
- Constipation
- Poor appetite
- Burning sensation in the epigastric part
- Belching and indigestion

Treatment:

1. Therapeutic Method: Sooth the liver to regulate the circulation of *qi*, promote blood circulation to remove blood stasis

2. Manipulations: An and Rou

3. Point Selection: Geshu (BL 17), Ganshu (BL 18), Danshu (BL 19), Jiuwei (RN 15), Zhangmen (LR 13), Dannang (EX-LE 6), and non-fixed points along the Bladder Channel in the back

4. Operation:

   a. The patient is prone. Stand to one side of the patient. Seek for the pressure pain points carefully along the Bladder Channel of Foot-Taiyang in the back, and press them gently with the right middle finger. At the same time, put the left middle finger on Jiuwei and apply An in an upward motion for two to three minutes. When the pain stops, gently An to Geshu, Danshu, and Ganshu three to five times each.

    b. The patient is supine. Sit at one side of the patient and apply An with the right middle finger to Zhangmen and Qimen (LR 14) for about two to three minutes until mild soreness occurs.

    c. The patient is supine. Conduct An with force on Dannang (both sides) with the surfaces of both thumbs. Repeat 50 times.

5. Supplement:

    a. In the case of nausea and inclination to vomit: Rou to Neiguan (PC 6) and Zhongwan (RN 12).

    b. In the case of radiating pain in the back and scapular region: Rou to Jianzhen (SI 9), Bingfeng (SI 12), and Jianjing (GB 21).

    c. In the case of constipation: Rou to Tianshu (ST 25) and Shenque (RN 8).

6. Treatment Course: Treatment is given once daily for six days.

Note: Persuade the patient to rest calmly and pay attention to changes in the patient's body temperature. When the condition grows worse, drugs should be given promptly.

6.15 Mastitis

Mastitis is common on postpartum lactation. Most subjects are primiparae.

Etiology and Pathology:

Mastitis is due to stagnation of both *qi* and blood caused by the following three factors:

1. Stagnancy of liver-*qi*

2. Accumulation of abundant stomach-heat

3. Noxious-fire may cause papillary destruction and/or galactostasis to invade the breasts

Clinical Manifestations:

1. Mastitis due to stagnation of liver-*qi*:

- Distending pain in the breast with tender mass but without red skin
- Irritability
- Bitter taste in the mouth
- Poor appetite
- Thin, white tongue coating
- Taut pulse

2. Mastitis due to stomach-heat:

- Red, swollen, burning and painful mammary mass that may lead to mammary swelling and masthelcosis
- Fever and aversion to cold
- Dry mouth and tongue
- Constipation
- Yellow tongue coating
- Taut, rapid, or slippery pulse.

Treatment:

Treatment differs according to the stage of the disease (initial, suppurative, or ulcerative stage). Tuina is usually given in the initial stage.

1. Therapeutic Method: Soothe the liver to regulate *qi* flow and relieve swelling to dredge the collaterals.

2. Manipulations: Mo, Mo, and Nieji

3. Point Selection: Rugen (ST 18), Ruzhong (ST 17), Qimen (LR 14), Danzhong (RN 17), Shaoze (SI 11), Hegu (LI 4), Ganshu (BL 18), Pishu (BL 20), and Weishu (BL 21)

4. Operation:

   a. The patient is supine. Sit on the side of the affected part.

      i. Rou with the thenar of one hand rapidly and moderately around the mass for five minutes.

      ii. Gently Nie (pinch) and Rou around the mass with both thumbs and index fingers.

      iii. Rou with the middle finger to Rugen, Ruzhong, and Qimen for one minute each.

   b. The patient is sitting. Sit face to face with the patient and spread talc powder on the affected part.

      i. Prop the breast with the left hand.

      ii. Lightly, gently, and rhythmically Nieji toward the nipple for two minutes with the thumb and index finger of the right hand, expelling the stagnated milk until yellowish milk is seen.

   c. The patient is prone. Stand at one side of the patient.

      i. Perform Tui with the surface of the thumb on Ganshu, Pishu, and Weishu for one minute each.

      ii. AnRou with the surface of the thumb on each side of Ganshu, Pishu, and Weishu. Repeat three to five times.

5. Treatment Course: Treatment is given once daily for three days.

Note: Be careful to keep the nipples clean. Additionally, the mouth cavity of the infant should be cleaned, and prompt treatment should be given to a cracked nipple. Remember that tuina is not used in the suppurative and ulcerative stages.

6.16 Dysmenorrhea

Dysmenorrhea is characterized by symptoms such as:
• Distending pain of the lower abdomen
• Soreness and weakness of the loins and knees especially before, after, or during the menstrual period. Severe cases disturb one's ability to work and lift.

Etiology and Pathology:
Mental disorders, an attack of exogenous cold pathogens, and a diet of cold food and drink leads to stagnation of *qi* and blood, causing dysmenorrhea.

Clinical Manifestations:
1. Dysmenorrhea due to stagnant *qi*:
• Tender and distended lower abdomen before or during menstruation
• Scanty menstruation or difficulty menstruating
• Distending pain in the breasts
• Headache or migraine
• Reddened tongue
• Deep and uneven pulse

2. Dysmenorrhea due to cold-dampness:
• Cold pain in the lower abdomen before or during the menstrual period
• Scanty, pale, or dark red menstrual blood with clots
• White, moist, and greasy tongue coating
• Deep and tense pulse

3. Dysmenorrhea due to deficient *qi* and blood:
• Dull pain relieved by pressing in the lower abdomen after the menstrual period
• Scanty, pale, and thin menstruation
• Lassitude
• Acratia

- Pale complexion
- Pale tongue with white coating
- Deep, thready, and weak pulse

Treatment:

1. Therapeutic Method: Activate *qi* flow to remove blood stasis, warm the channels to dispel cold, and replenish *qi* to nourish blood.

2. Manipulations: Yizhichan Tui, An, Mo, and Ca

3. Point Selection: Suliao (DU 25), Guanyuan (RN 4), Qihai (RN 6), Shenshu (BL 23), Baliao (BL 31-34), Hegu (LI 4), and Sanyinjiao (SP 6)

4. Operation:

   a. The patient is supine.

      i. Mo with the palm on the lower abdomen for about seven to eight minutes until the patient has a hot sensation.

      ii. AnRou to either Qihai or Guanyuan three to five times.

      iii. Rou to Suliao at the tip of the nose for one minute.

   b. The patient is prone.

      i. DiAn-An to Baliao with both hands for about three minutes.

      ii. Ca with the hypothenar to Baliao.

      iii. An to Shenshu.

   c. Qia to either Hegu or Sanyinjiao for about two minutes.

5. Supplement:

   a. In the case of deficient *qi*: Mo to the abdomen counterclockwise

   b. In the case of stagnant *qi*: Mo to the abdomen clockwise.

   c. In the case of nausea with tendency to vomit: Tui to Zhongwan (RN 12), Neiguan (PC 6), and Danzhong (RN 17).

   d. In the case of stagnant liver-*qi*: AnRou to Ganshu (BL 18) and Qimen (LR 14).

6. Treatment Course: Treatment is given once daily for six days.

6.17 Postpartum General Aching

Soreness and numbness of the limbs after giving birth is called postpartum general aching.

Etiology and Pathology:
Pain is caused by the obstruction of channels due to:
- Inability of blood to nourish the muscles and tendons due to postpartum deficient *qi* blood
- Invasion of wind-cold-dampness

Clinical Manifestations:
1. Aching due to weakness of *qi* and blood:
   - Soreness and numbness of the limbs
   - Pale complexion
   - Pale tongue with a slight coating
   - Thready and weak pulse
2. Aching due to exogenous wind-cold-dampness:
   - Migrating pain or heavy sensation and swelling in the limbs
   - Pale tongue with thin white coating
   - Thready and rapid pulse

Treatment:
1. Therapeutic Method: Nourish *qi* and blood, warm the channels, and dispel cold.
2. Manipulations: An, Rou, Qia, and Na
3. Point Selection: Jianjing (GB 21), Pishu (BL 20), Weishu (BL 21), Shenshu (BL 23), Shousanli (LI 10, Neiguan (PC 6), Waiguan (SJ 5), Hegu (LI 4), Quchi (LI 11), Zusanli (ST 36), and Chengshan (BL 57)
4. Operation:
   a. The patient is prone.
      i. AnRou to Pishu, Weishu, and Shenshu for about three minutes.
      ii. Gentle Gun from the top to bottom of the legs for two to three minutes.
      iii. An to Zusanli three to five times.
      iv. Na to Chengshan three to five times.
   b. The patient is sitting.
      i. Qia and Rou to Shousanli, Quchi, Neiguan, Waiguan, Waiguan, Hegu, and Jianjing for about five minutes
      ii. Na to Jianjing two to three times.
5. Treatment Course: Treatment is given once daily for five days.

6.18 Postpartum Tormina

Postpartum tormina is pain in the lower abdomen after giving birth.

Etiology and Pathology:

Postpartum tormina is due to either of the following:

- Blood stasis resulting from weakened *qi* and blood in the Chong and Ren channels
- Stagnated blood resulting from the invasion of pathogenic cold and from weakened *qi* and blood

Clinical Manifestations:

1. Due to deficient blood:

- Dull pain relieved by pressing the lower abdomen
- Small and pale lochia
- Dizziness
- Blurred vision
- Pale nails and complexion
- Constipation
- Lassitude
- Acratia
- Pale tongue with a thin coating
- Deficient, thready, and weak pulse

2. Due to blood stasis:

- Pain relieved by warmth but aggravated by pressing the lower abdomen
- Cold limbs
- Small lochia with blood stasis
- Dark purple tongue with white, slippery coating
- Deep and uneven pulse

3. Due to accumulation of cold:

- Cold pain relieved by either pressing or warmth
- Cold limbs
- Small lochia
- Dark, pale tongue with white and slippery coating
- Deep and tense pulse

Treatment:

1. Therapeutic Method: Strengthen *qi* and blood, promote blood circulation to remove blood stasis, and warm the channels to dispel cold.

2. Manipulations: Mo, An, Rou, and Ca

3. Point Selection: Guanyuan (RN 4), Shimen (RN 5), Sanyinjiao (SP 6), Dahe (KI 12), Pishu (BL 20), Shenshu (BL 23), Mingmen (DU 4), Baliao (BL 31-34), and Shiqizhui (EX-B 8)

4. Operation:

   a. The patient is supine.

       i. Mo over the lower abdomen for about five minutes.

       ii. An to Guanyuan, Shimen, Sanyinjiao, and Dahe for two minutes.

   b. The patient is prone.

       i. Rou with fingers on Pishu, Shenshu, Mingmen, Baliao, and Shiqizhui for about five minutes.

       ii. Ca with palms on Baliao until the patient feels a hot sensation.

5. Treatment Course: Treatment is given once daily for seven days.

6.19 Toothache

According to western medicine, a toothache is a symptom of dental cavities, pulpitis, and periodontitis.

Etiology and Pathology:

According to TCM, the consumption of too much pungent and greasy food leads to production of stomach-heat. Prolonged accumulation of stomach-heat turns into fire, and fire tends to go up to cause swelling and pain in the gums. Toothaches can also be caused by fire of the deficiency type due to insufficient kidney-*yin*.

Clinical Manifestations:

1. Due to stomach-fire:

   • Severe toothache

   • Foul breath

   • Constipation

   • Yellow and greasy tongue coating

   • Rapid and forceful pulse

2. Due to wind-fire:
- Severe pain with swelling
- Cold limbs
- Floating pulse

3. Due to deficient kidney-*yin*:
- Intermittent dull pain
- Loose teeth
- Thready pulse

Treatment:

1. Therapeutic Method: Remove heat from the stomach to clear away fire, expel wind to dispel heat, and nourish *yin* to sweep away fire.

2. Manipulations: An, Rou, Qia, Nie, and Na

3. Point Selection: Jiache (ST 6), Xiaguan (ST 7), Neiting (SI 44), Hegu (LI 4), Waiguan (SJ 5), Fengchi (GB 20), Taixi (KI 3), and Xingjian (LR 2)

4. Operation:

   a. The patient is sitting. Stand at one side of the patient and fix his/her head with the left hand.

      i. An to Jiache and Xiaguan with the right hand for two to three minutes.

      ii. Rou on Jiache and Xiaguan for two to three minutes.

   b. The patient is sitting. Stand to the side of the patient. Na with the right hand to each side of Hegu for one to two minutes. This should relieve the pain right away. If pain of the right side is severe, treat the right side first.

   c. The patient sits with his/her legs stretched out. Qia to Neiting, Taixi, or Xingjian.

5. Treatment Course: Treatment is given once daily for three days.

6.20 Pharyngitis

Characteristics of pharyngitis include dry throat, pharyngolynia, and pharyngeal paraesthesia.

Etiology and Pathology:

Two types of pharyngitis are:
- Throat pain of the excess type: Exogenous wind-heat burns the lung or stomach system and rises in both channels

- Throat pain of deficiency type: Fire of deficiency type due to deficient kidney-*yin*

Clinical Manifestations:

1. Due to excess heat:

- Sore throat
- Dry mouth with desire for drink
- Foul breath
- Swollen gums
- Burning pain in the epigastric region
- Deep red tongue with yellow, greasy coating
- Slippery and rapid pulse

2. Due to *yin*-deficiency:

- Dry and itchy throat
- Low and hoarse voice
- Thirst with desire for drink
- Cough without or with a little sputum
- Reddened tongue without or with a slight coating
- Thready and rapid pulse

Treatment:

1. Therapeutic Method: Clear away heat to relieve sore throat and nourish *yin* to expel fire.

2. Manipulations: Na, Rou, and Qia

3. Point Selection: Fengchi (GB 20), Tianzhu (BL 10), Renying (ST 9), Lianquan (RN 23), Quchi (LI 11), Hegu (LI 4), Shaoshang (LU 11), and Shangyang (LI 1)

4. Operation:

   a. The patient is sitting. Stand behind the patient and support his/her forehead with your left hand.

      i. Na to Fengchi and Tianzhu with the thumb and the index finger of the right hand for about four to five minutes until the patient feels increased secretion in the mouth.

      ii. Rou gently to Renying and Lianquan for about two minutes.

   b. Qiarou to Quchi, Hegu, Shaoshang, and Shangyang for about five minutes.

5. Supplement:

   a. In the case of deficient kidney-*qi*: Qiarou to Taixi (KI 3) and Zhaohai (LI 6).

b. In the case of constipation due to abundant heat in the lung and stomach: Qiarou Fenglong (ST 40) and Zhigou (SJ 6).

6. Treatment course: Treatment is given once daily for three days.

6.21 Dislocation of Tendon of Long Head of Biceps Brachii

The long tendon of the brachia biceps starts from the superior node of the pelvis of scapula, stretches downward to pass over the head of humerus and through the superior transverse ligament of scapula and the tendon sheath of the brachia biceps, and enters the osseofibrous canal of intertubercular sulcus. Under normal conditions, the movement of the shoulder causes this long tendon of the brachial biceps to slide longitudinally but not to the right or left.

Etiology and Pathology:

The tendon shifts into medial side, or out, of the intertubercular sulcus when laceration and dislocation of the soft tissues protecting the long tendon of the biceps (See Figure 81). Laceration and/or dislocation occur if the arm is over-abducted or outwardly rotated and one of the following conditions exists:

- Flaccid superior transverse ligament of scapula
- Flaccid or prolonged long tendon of the biceps
- Shallow bed of the bottom of the intertubercular sulcus
- Congenital abnormal development of the microjoints
- Lessened slope of the medial wall of the intertubercular sulcus
- Local retrograde affection and hyperosteogeny
- Laceration of the superior transverse ligament of scapula
- Acute or chronic laceration or dislocation of the end of either the greater pectoral muscle or the subscapular muscle (due to trauma of the shoulder)

Clinical Manifestations:

Dislocation of tendon of long head of biceps brachii falls into two categories in clinical practice: habitual and traumatic. The former is chronic but usually due to mild trauma that easily relapses. Acute dislocation due to trauma is marked by the following abrupt symptoms and signs:

- Pain in the anterior of the shoulder
- Inwardly rotated humerus
- Dysfunction of the joint in abduction, adduction, outward-rotation, and inward-rotation

- Arm failing to swing forward and backward; patient often has to prop it with his/her other hand when walking to lessen the pain caused by the arm's swinging movement

Treatment:

Tuina is effective in treating both habitual and traumatic dislocation of tendon of long head of biceps brachii. However, even with tuina therapy, habitual dislocation tends to relapse. Therefore, suture, if necessary, should be performed.

Tuina is much more effective in the treatment of traumatic dislocation except when the traumatic dislocation of the tendon is due to a dislocation of the shoulder or fracture of humeral neck; in this case, orthopedia taxis is needed.

1. Therapeutic Method: Restore and treat injured soft tissues, dredge the channels, and promote blood circulation.

2. Manipulations: Yizhichan Tui, Rou, Cuo, and Bashen

3. Point Selection: Jianyu (LI 15), Jianjing (GB 21), Binao (LI 14), Quchi (LI 11), Shousanli (LI 10), Waiguan (SJ 5), and Hegu (LI 4)

4. Operation:

   a. The patient is sitting. Stand in front of the patient, and put four fingers of the right hand on the affected shoulder of the patient with the palm downward and the thumb on the midpoint of the anterior border of the deltoid muscle (where the tendon of long head of biceps brachii is located). Firmly support the neck of the humerus; with the left hand, hold the wrist of the affected arm with the patient's palm forward and shoulder 60 abducted and 40 forward-flexed.

   b. While doing counter-traction with both hands, rotate the forearm of the patient progressively backward until the shoulder is 40 abducted and the lowered forearm is rotated as far back as possible. At the same time, push the right thumb outward and upward to firmly press the dislocated tendon of long head of the biceps brachii. Rotate

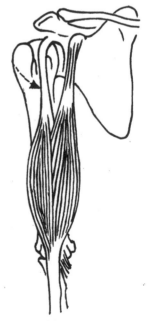

Figure 81

the affected arm rapidly forward with the left hand (See Figure 82).

c. Using your thumb, push and knead gently the tendon of long head of biceps brachii for three to five minutes. Then conduct gentle Cuo and Rou around the shoulder with both palms. If necessary, keep the affected arm in the position of adduction and intorsion suspended for two to four weeks. Then move the shoulder properly lest local adhesion occur.

5. Treatment Course: Treatment is given once daily for three days.

6.22 Tenosynovitis of Long Head of Biceps Brachii

When the shoulder is abducted or rotated outward, the tendon of long head of the biceps brachii slides in the greatest amplitude within its tendon sheath.

Etiology and Pathology:

Inflammation caused by:

- Repeated friction between the tendon and the tendon sheath due to prolonged and powerful abduction or outward rotation of the shoulder

- Injury due to sudden traction. In this case, the tendon sheath shows dropsy, degeneration, thickness, roughness, and/or fibrosis; occasionally the fiber between the tendon sheath and the tendon adheres.

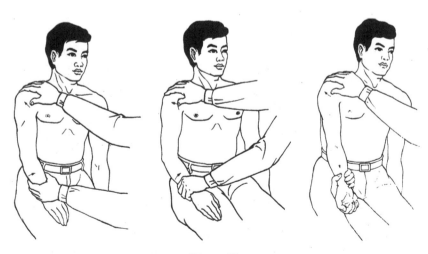

Figure 82

Clinical Manifestations:
Generally, patients will exhibit the following indications:
- Local pain radiating to the inferior of the deltoid muscle
- Severe tenderness in the tendon of long head of the biceps brachii
- Limited joint movement
- Mild rubbing sensation, often felt when the biceps muscle of arm is being diastolized and contracted
- Pain, especially when the patient lifts things or contracts his/her biceps muscle

In cases due to chronic strain:
- Pressure point pain restricted to the intertubercular sulcus
- Pain occurring only when the shoulder is abducted and extended backward (usually not when movement in other direction is being done).

Treatment:
Rapid curative effects are attained when tuina is used to treat cases due to acute trauma. A longer course of tuina treatment is needed to treat cases due to chronic strain. During treatment, reduce the movement of the affected shoulder, especially active abduction.

1. Therapeutic Method: Relax the tendon, dredge the collaterals, remove blood stasis, and relieve pain.

2. Manipulations: Yizhichan Tui, Tanbo, Rou, Ca, Yao, and Dou

3. Point Selection: Jianneiling, Jianyu (LI 15), Jianjing (GB 21), and Binao (LI 14)

4. Operation:

   a. The patient is sitting. Stand or sit to the affected side of the patient, and use the edge or belly of the thumb to conduct Yizhichan Tui for three to five minutes from the tendon of long head of the biceps brachii to the intertubercular sulcus, where the point Jianneiling is located.

   b. With your thumb, gently conduct Tanbo on the tendon of long head of the biceps brachii 20-30 times. Gently perform Na downward along the deltoid muscle up to the elbow.

   c. Put both palms on the affected shoulder with one at the anterior and the other at the posterior. Perform Cuo in opposite directions for about one to two minutes. Then rotate the shoulder clockwise for three circles and counterclockwise for three circles. Finally, Dou the arm.
   As an alternative, you can apply Chinese ilex ointment to the shoulder, and conduct Ca in the direction towards the inter-

turbercular sulcus with the hypothenar up to the extent that the heat produced goes deep. Add a hot compress to intensify the effect.

5. Treatment Course: Treatment is given once daily for five days.

6.23 Tendinitis of Supraspinatus Muscle

Supraspinous muscle, part of rotator cuff, starts from the supraspinous fossa of the scapula. Its tendon goes from under acromial tendon of coracoid process and subacromial bura to above the narrow space superior to shoulder capsule. It terminates at the superior of the greater tuberosity of humerus, connecting closely with the joint capsule to increase its stability. Supraspinous muscle allows the upper arm to abduct.

Etiology and Pathology:

Prolonged and repeated abduction of the arm tends to injure the tendon of supraspinous muscle or to lead to chronic strain and degeneration of the tendon, causing an aseptic inflammation.

Clinical Manifestations:

This disorder is marked by pain, tenderness, and limited abduction.

- Pain at the lateral aspect of the shoulder. The pain usually spreads to the attachment of the deltoid muscle and sometimes radiates up the neck and down the elbow, forearm, and fingers.

- Tenderness at the greater tubercle where the tendon of supraspinous muscle terminates.
  Tenderness can turn to severe pain when the shoulder is 60 - 120 abducted, and muscle atrophy may be seen in prolonged cases.

Treatment:

Tuina is very effective in treating this disease. If the tendonitis is in the acute stage, apply the manipulations gently and slowly, and restrict movement of the shoulder. If it is in the chronic stage, apply the manipulations with a deepening effect. Supplement tuina manipulations with exercise and heat/warmth.

1. Therapeutic Method: Promote blood circulation to remove blood stasis and expel obstruction in the channels and collaterals.

2. Manipulations: Yizhichan Tui, An, Rou, Na, Pingtui (flat-push), Yao, and Dou

3. Point Selection: Jianjing (GB 21), Bingfeng (SI 12), Quyuan (SI 13), Tianzong (SI 11), Jianwaishu (SI 14), Naoshu (SI 10), and Binao (LI 14)

4. Operation

   a. The patient is sitting. Stand to the affected side of the patient, passively (with the muscles relaxed) abduct the affected arm 30 and prop the patient's elbow with your hand. For three to five minutes, apply Yizhichan Tui to and fro at the top of the subacromial greater tuberosity of humerus and along the suprospinous muscle.

   b. Alternately conduct Tanbo and AnRou with the thumb over the affected portion for three to five minutes.

   c. Apply some ointment made from Chinese holly leaf to the part where the supraspinous muscle of scapula is located. Perform Pingtui with the palm root or hypothenar. At the same time, DiAn-An with the tip of the middle or index finger on the points Bingfeng, Quyuan, Jianwaishu, and Jianliao (SJ 14). Pingtui should be done to the extent that hot sensation is deepening, while with DiAn-An until soreness and distention occur.

   d. NieNa Jianjing and the deltoid muscle three to five times.

   e. Rotate the shoulder clockwise three times and counterclockwise three times; CuoRou the affected arm three to five times to and fro from the shoulder to the wrist, and, finally, Doula the affected arm.

   Local hot compress may be added during the treatment.

5. Treatment course: Treatment is given once daily for three days.

6.24 Subacromial Bursitis

There are many synovial bursae around the shoulder, the largest of which are the subacromial bursa and the subdeltoid bursa. The former is below the acromion, and the latter is on the deep part of the deltoid muscle. They function mainly in preventing friction between the greater tuberosity of humerus and the acromial process.

Etiology and Pathology:

Acute traumatic subacromial bursitis is caused by injury of the synovial bursae in the deep layer of the deltoid muscle due to direct or indirect trauma of the shoulder, while chronic subacromial bursitis is due to degeneration of the synovial bursae. In addition, degeneration of the synovial bursa due to prolonged repeated strain leads to aseptic inflammation marked by bursal edema and thickness or adhesion of the bursal walls. Both symptoms limit abduction and rotation of the arm and normal function of the shoulder.

Clinical Manifestations:

Pain on the lateral aspect of the shoulder often radiates to the end of the deltoid muscle and becomes severe when the arm is abducted or rotated to the outside. Additional manifestations include:

- Tenderness in the subacromial region
- Round mass on the anterior border of the deltoid muscle appearing in the acute stage due to bursal tympany
- Slightly restricted shoulder movement that becomes progressively limited because of adhesion of rotator cuff
- Atrophy of the supraspinous and infraspinous muscles and, later, the deltoid muscle

Treatment:

Perform treatment with gentle manipulations during the acute stage. Be sure not to press the affected area hard lest the injury of the bursa be worsened. During this stage, the patient need not limit his/her shoulder movement.

During the chronic stage, apply more powerful manipulations, prescribe appropriate functional exercises for the patient to perform regularly, and keep the affected part warm.

1. Therapeutic Method: In the acute stage, remove blood stasis to relieve pain. In the chronic stage, promote blood circulation to remove blood stasis and lubricate the joint.

2. Manipulations: Yizhichan Tui, Rou, Cuo, Pingtui, Dou, and Yao

3. Point Selection: Jianyu (LI 15), Binao (LI 14), Jianneiling, Tianzong (SI 11), and Quchi (LI 11)

4. Operation:

    a. The patient is sitting. Stand to the affected side of the patient, and Yizhichan Tui to and fro around the deltoid for three to five minutes.

    b. Apply ointment of the Chinese holly leaf or oil of safflower to the lateral, anterior, and posterior aspects of the arm. Pingtui until the heat produced goes deep. Then hold the arm with both hands, and CuoRou with both palms to and fro along the upper arm and forearm three to five times.

    c. AnRou with the tip of the thumb or the middle finger on Tianzong, Jianyu, Quchi, Shousanli (LI 10), and Hegu (LI 4) until the patient feels sore and distending.

    d. Yao the affected arm gently in a circle and gently DouLa the affected arm.

    e. To decrease inflammation, add hot compress locally after the manipulations.

5. Treatment course: Treatment is given once daily for five days.

6.25 External Humeral Epicondylitis

Common in middle-aged people, this disorder is also called tennis elbow and humeroradial bursistis.

Etiology and Pathology:

The external humeral epicondyle is the place on which the brachioradial muscle and the general tendon of the forearm extensor are fixed. If the wrist is dorsi-extended often when the forearm is in the pronator position, the soft tissues near the point of attachment can be injured. This causes pulls, local bleeding, adhesion, and even pain due to invasion of the joint synovium into the humeroradial articulation. In absence of evident trauma, humeroradial bursistis is usually due to either acute sprain or chronic strain. It is common in middle-aged patients who repeatedly rotate their forearms and stretch their wrists strenuously.

Clinical Manifestations:

Soreness on the lateral aspect of the elbow's posterior worsens when rotating and extending, lifting, pulling, holding, or pushing. The soreness radiates downward along the extensor muscle of wrist, and the following additional manifestations occur

- Local mild swelling

- Difficulty in rotating the forearm and holding things

Treatment:

Good results are attained with tuina manipulations, especially in cases with short disease duration. If cases of longer duration fail to respond to tuina treatment, operation should be considered.

1. Therapeutic Method: Relax the muscles and tendons, remove obstruction from the channels, and promote blood circulation to eliminate blood stasis.

2. Manipulations: Yizhichan Tui, Rou, Tanbo, and Ca

3. Point Selection: Quchi (LI 11), humeroradial articulation space, shousanli (LI 10), Waiguan (SJ 5), and Hegu (LI 4)

4. Operation:

    a. Sit to the affected side of the patient in the sitting position. Yizhichan Tui to and fro from the external humeral epicondyle to the forearm three to five minutes. Tanbo locally five to ten times.

b. Tui on the affected side. For the right side, hold the wrist of the patient with your right hand and rotate his/her right forearm to the supinator position. Press the anterior of the external humeral epicondyle with your flexed left thumb, and put the other four fingers on the medial aspect of the elbow. With your right hand, flex the patient's elbow gradually to the maximum. With your left thumb, press hard on the anterior of the patient's external humeral epicondyle and straighten the bent elbow. At the same time, shift your left thumb to the anterior and superior of the affected radial head and conduct backward Tanbo on the origin of the wrist extensor muscle along the anterior-lateral border of the radial head. (For treatment to the left side, reverse the hands with which you hold the patient and perform the manipulations.)

c. Apply Chinese holly leaf ointment or safflower oil to the elbow's lateral aspect. Pingtui the external humeral epicondyle and the forearm's extensor muscles until the heat produced goes deep. With your left hand, hold the far end of the humerus and Dou the forearm and elbow.

5. Treatment Course: Treatment is given once daily for seven days.

6.26 Medial Humeral Epicondylitis

Medial humeral epicondylitis is also called "student elbow," for it is common in youth and young children.

Etiology and Pathology:

The medial humeral epicondyle is the attachment of the general tendon of forearm flexor.

- Prolonged and repeated wrist flexion, wrist extension, and forearm pronation result in strain of the medial humeral epicondyle attachment, which leads to chronic aseptic inflammation.

- Acute laceration occurs at the attachment point of tendon due to traumatic injury, dorsoextension of the wrist, and abduction and pronation of the forearm. Acute laceration promotes hematoma and fibrosis and causes strain of the medial humeral epicondyle.

Clinical Manifestations:

Soreness in and around the medial humeral epicondyle becomes more evident when the forearm is pronated or the wrist is actively flexed. The soreness radiates downward along the ulnar wrist flexor and manifests as follows:

- Difficulty in flexing the wrist
- Tenderness in the medial humeral epicondyle
- Extensive tenderness in the ulnar flexor and the superficial flexor of finger

Treatment:

1. Therapeutic Method: Relax muscles and tendons, eliminate obstruction from channels, and promote blood circulation to remove blood stasis.

2. Manipulations: An, Rou, Tanbo, Na, and CuoRou

3. Point Selection: Shaohai (HT 3), Xiaohai (SI 8), and Waiguan (SJ 5)

4. Operation:

   a. The patient is sitting. With your thumb, gently AnRou along the ulnar wrist flexor from the medial humeral epi-condyle to the wrist. At the same time, extend and flex the wrist to relax the tense wrist flexors.

   b. Tanbo at the pain pressure point in the medial humeral epicondyle and in the region around the point for two to three minutes. Gently and rapidly Na to and fro along the wrist flexor several times.

   c. With both palms, CuoRou the patient's elbow and the forearm. Then DouLa his/her forearm and elbow.

   d. Finally, apply Chinese holly leaf ointment to the medial humeral epicondyle and conduct local Ca and Mo until the heat produced goes deep.

5. Treatment Course: Treatment is given once daily for seven days.

6.27 Sprained Wrist

Including radiocarpal articulation and intercarpal joint, the wrist flexes, extends, adducts, abducts, and rotates. Sprains happen easily because of the wrist's broad and frequent movement.

Etiology and Pathology:

Injury of the soft tissues around the wrist is due to direct or indirect violence, overstrain due to overload or prolonged and repeated taxing work.

Clinical Manifestations:

A sprained wrist may or may not have evident trauma history. Pain on the dorsum when palm-flexing the wrist indicates injury to the dorsal carpal ligament and extensor digitorum. Pain that occurs regardless of the direction the wrist moves indicates a compound injury of the ligament and the tendon. The symptoms of an acute sprain are:

- Swelling and pain in the wrist
- Limited wrist function
- Pain that becomes severe when the wrist moves
- Local tenderness

The symptoms of a chronic sprain are:
- Mild pain in the wrist
- No evident swelling and distending
- Pain in the injured point when the joint moves in wide range
- Acratia and stiffness in the wrist
- Otherwise, the pain indicates injury to the ligamentum carpivolare or the tendon of the flexor.

Better curative effects will be attained if Tuina is used to treat sprained wrist.

Note: Many of the above symptoms are indicative of several different wrist disorders. In clinical practice, wrist sprain must be distinguished from the following disorders (which are treated through orthopedic reduction or operation):

- Fracture of the distal end of radius and ulna
- Fracture of scaphoid
- Fracture or dislocation of lunate bone
- Avulsion fracture of the dorsal aspect of triangular bone
- Aseptic necrosis of scaphoid and lunate bone

Treatment:

1. Therapeutic Method: Relax muscles and tendons, promote blood circulation, remove blood stasis, and relieve pain.
2. Manipulations: Yizhichan Tui, DiAn, An, Rou, Na, Ca, Tanjin (flicking), Yao, and Bashen
3. Point Selection: Shaohai (HT 3), Tongli (HT 5), Shenmen (HT 7), Chize (LU 57), Lieque (LU 7), Taiyuan (LU 9), Hegu (LI 4), Yangxi (LI 5), and Quchi (LI 11)
4. Operation:

Before beginning manipulations, select proper points around the injury and along the corresponding channels. As examples:

- Points along the Heart Channel of Hand-Shaoyin such as Shaohai, Tongli, and Shenmen may be selected on the ulnar palmar surface

- Points along the Lung Channel of Hand-Taiyin such as Chize, Lieque, and Taiyuan may be selected on the radial palmar surface

- Points along the Large Intestine Channel of Hand-Yangming such as Hegu, Yangxi, and Quchi may be selected on the radial dorsal surface

Select points in other regions in the same manner as the above.

Once you select the points, use gentle and slow manipulations to treat an acute injury that shows evident pain and swelling. After manipulations, prescribe hot compresses with herbal medicine to patients with distinct swelling.

a. DiAn, An, and Rou with the thumb until sensation of soreness and distension occurs. To promote the *qi* flow and blood through the channels and collaterals, continue the manipulations for another minute.

b. Yizhichan Tui—up, down, left, and right—around the injury for about three to five minutes. This action promotes blood circulation, removes blood stasis, and improves the blood circulation around the injury. Add the manipulations Na and Tanjin to relieve spasm.

c. Conduct Yao together with Bashen to enable the wrist to normally circle, dorsi-flex, palmar-flex and laterally-bend.

d. Apply safflower oil on the wrist and perform Ca until the heat produced goes deep.
When performing the manipulations, add appropriate pressure and increase the amplitude gradually to relieve the spasm, release the adhesion, and improve joint function.

5. Treatment Course: Treatment is given once daily for three days.

6.28 Carpal Tunnel Syndrome

Carpal tunnel syndrome is due to the median nerve being pressed within the carpal canal.

Etiology and Pathology:

Transverse palmar ligaments and carpal bone form a carpal canal. The transverse palmar ligaments are on the palmar surface, and the carpal bone is on the posterior. Besides the median nerve, the carpal canal includes four tendons of the superficial flexor muscle of fingers, four tendons of the deep flexor muscle of fingers, and one tendon of the long flexor muscle of thumb. As tendons in the carpal canal enlarge, the tendons and median nerve press against each other and nervous symp-

toms appear. Related disorders include hyperplasia, fracture and dislocation of carpal bone, pachynsis of interosseous intercarpal ligaments, and
swelling and distension of the tendons in the carpal canal.

Clinical Manifestations:

1. In the initial stage:

 * Finger numbness and pain that is stabbing and that often
disturbs sleep but is relieved as soon as the affected hand is
waved

 * Numbness and pain of the index, middle, and ring fingers and
the thumb but not of the little finger

 * Burning pain of the small finger in a few cases

2. In the later stage:

 * Atrophy

 * Numbness and myodynamic attenuation of the thenar eminence muscles (short abductor muscle of thumb and opposing
muscle of thumb)

 * Semi-radial anesthesia of the thumb and the index, middle,
and ring fingers

 * Myophagism gradually appearing four months after the onset

 * Hypoesthesia or anesthesia of the fingers with the symptoms
found in examination

 * Pain in the palm that does not go away

 * Symptoms aggravated if the point Daling (PC 7) is pressed on
the affected limb

Treatment:

Tuina is only suitable for carpal tunnel syndrome due to tendon
tumefaction resulting from injury or diseases. Operation is applicable to
other forms of carpal tunnel.

1. Therapeutic method: Relax muscles and tendons, eliminate
obstruction from the channels and collaterals, and promote
blood circulation to remove blood stasis.

2. Manipulations: Yizhichan Tui, An, Rou, Yao, and Ca

3. Point Selection: Quze (PC 3), Neiguan (PC 6), and Daling
(PC 7)

4. Operation:

 a. The patient is sitting upright. Sit next to the patient and
extend his/her hand, palm upward. Prop the dorsum of
his/her wrist with one hand and AnRou with the other hand
on the points Quze, Neiguan, Daling, and Yuji (LU 10).

b. Gently Yizhichan Tui to and fro from the forearm to the hand along the Pericardium Channel of Hand-Jueyin for three to five minutes. Concentrate on the area including the carpal canal and the thenar eminence. Gradually add pressure as you perform Yizhichan Tui.

Next, YaoRou the wrist and interphalangeal articulations of hand. Then Ca the carpometacarpus to relax the wrists' muscles and tendons, eliminate obstruction from the channels and collaterals, and promote blood circulation to remove blood stasis.

c. The patient is sitting upright. Place the patient's forearm in the pronator position with the dorsum of the hand upward. Hold the patient's palm with both of your hands as follows: Right hand on the radial aspect, left hand on the ulnar aspect, your thumbs flat on the dorsum of the wrist, and the tips of your thumbs pressed into the space on the dorsal aspect of the wrist. Perform Niewan.

Yao the wrist while Bashen is being done. Then dorsi-extend the wrist pressed by the thumbs to the maximum, flex it and circle it clockwise two to three times and counterclockwise two to three times as well (See Figure 83).

Following the manipulations, apply an ointment that warms the channels and dredges the collaterals to the wrist. The patient should keep the wrist in a resting position. Fumigate and wash with a decoction of herbal medicines after the symptoms are relieved.

5. Treatment Course: Treatment is given once daily for ten days.

6.29 Injury of Medial or Lateral Accessory Ligament of the Knee

The medial accessory ligament connects the medial condyle of the femur and the medial condyle of tibia like a bridge. Its medial aspect closely attaches to the lateral border of the medial and the posterior portion of medial semilunar plate. While the knee extends and flexes,

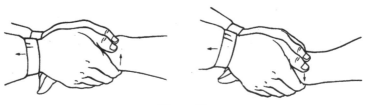

Figure 83

the ligament slides forward and backward on the medial condyle of femur.

When the knee extends or flexes completely, the ligament is tense. When the knee partially flexes, the ligament loosens, making the joint unstable and easy to injure.

Etiology and Pathology:

Sudden stress of inversion or extension to a partially flexed or extended knee can injure the medial or external accessory ligament.

Clinical Manifestations:

Sprain or partial laceration of the medial accessory ligament:

• History of trauma, pain and tenderness on the medial aspect of the knee; the pain becomes severe when the shank is passively abducted

• Local edema on the medial aspect of the knee

• Ecchymoses and hematocele within the knee may appear within two to three days after the onset

Complete rupture of the medial accessory ligament:

• Space (noticeable to the touch) in the broken ligament

• Abnormal "outward-turning" of the knee

• Avulsion of selerite seen in the ligament's end,

• Obviously widened medial space (compared with the normal side) seen in the X-ray

Treatment:

Tuina is usually suitable for the treatment of sprain and partial laceration of ligament. To treat complete rupture of ligament, operative suture or neoplasty should be given as soon as possible.

1. Therapeutic Method: Promote blood circulation to remove blood stasis, relieve swelling, and alleviate pain.

2. Manipulations: DiAn, An, Yizhichan Tui, Rou, Mo, and Pingtui

3. Point Selection: Ashi points around the injury, Xuehai (SP 10), Sanyinjiao (SP 6), Yinlingquan (SP 9), Xiguan (LR 7), and Ququan (LR 8)

4. Operation:

   a. The patient is supine with his/her injured limb straightened and outwardly rotated. DiAn on the points Xuehai, Yinlingquan, and Sanyinjiao to promote *qi* flow and blood through the channels and collaterals and to relieve pain.

   b. Gently and locally Rou with the palm or thenar eminence for three to five minutes. Then gently Yizhichan Tui with the thumb up and down along the medial accessory ligament for three to five minutes. Gradually increase the pressure of Yizhichan Tui over the course of the three-to-five minutes.

c. Coat the manipulated part with Chinese holly leaf ointment or safflower oil and Pingtui until the heat produced goes deep.
Fresh injury with evident pain should be treated with gentle manipulations and older injuries with stronger ones.
Note: Rare in clinical practice, injury of lateral accessory ligament is manifested and treated similarly to that of the medial accessory ligament.

5. Treatment Course: Treatment is given once daily for three days.

6.30 Sprained Ankle

The ankle is a hinge joint made up of the lower ends of the tibia and fibula and the talus. Its capsule is lax in the anterior and posterior but tense on both sides. It has thinner and weaker ligaments in the anterior and posterior, but stronger accessory ligaments on the medial and lateral sides.

Etiology and Pathology:

When the metatarsus flexes, the posterior portion of talus enters the ankle and makes unsteady. If the foot turns inward or outward suddenly while the ankle is in this unsteady state, either the lateral collateral ligament or the medial collateral ligament stresses and causes the sprained ankle.

Clinical Manifestations:

- History of acute sprain
- Evident ankle swelling and pain that worsens when the patient stands
- Tenderness in the antero-inferior of both the medial and lateral malleoli
- Purple (bruised-like) skin
- Sprain of lateral malleolus marked by pain in the lateral ankle; the pain becomes aggravated when the ankle turns inward
- Swelling and distention in the lateral joint and the anteroinferior of lateral malleolus when the lateral joint capsule and anterior fibula ligament are injured
- Possible fracture of the lateral malleolus following a sprain of medial malleolus

Treatment:

Better effects will be attained if tuina manipulations are used to treat simple sprain of ligament or laceration of partial ligamentous fibrae. If a sprain is accompanied by a fracture or dislocation, orthopedic operation or manula reduction should be performed as early as possible.

1. Therapeutic Method: Promote blood circulation to remove blood stasis, relieve swelling, and alleviate pain.

2. Manipulations: DiAn, An, Yizhichan Tui, Rou, Bashen, and Yao

3. Point Selection: Ashi points around the ankle, Zusanli (ST 36), Yanglingquan (GB 34), Taixi (KI 3), Kunlun (BL 60), Qiuxu (GB 40), Xuanzhong (GB 39), Jiexi (ST 41), and Taichong (LR 3)

4. Operation:

   a. The patient is supine. DiAn the points Zusanli, Taixi, Kunlun, Qiuxu, Zuanzhong, Jiexi, and Taichong to remove obstruction from the channels and collaterals and to relieve pain.

   b. Locally Rou with the thenar for three to five minutes, and then Tui with the thumb from top to bottom over the shank and around the ankle. This manipulation promotes blood circulation, removes blood stasis, relieves swelling, and alleviates pain.

   c. The patient is supine. Tightly hold the patient's big toe on the affected foot and pull it upward. Turn the ankle outward to enlarge its medial space, and press your left index finger into the space. Turn the ankle inward while keeping the traction to enlarge the ankle's lateral space, and press the left thumb into the space. Hold the ankle with the thumb and index finger, and gently pull and shake the affected foot. Turn the ankle inward one to two times with the right hand. Dorsi- and plantar flex the foot, and push down and pull up both the medial and lateral malleoli while holding the ankle with your thumb and index finger. Make sure that the push follows the dorsi-flexion and the pull follows the plantar-flexion (See Figure 84).

   d. If muscular spasm and adhesion accompany the sprained ankle, do the following: Hold the Achilles tendon with one hand and the big toe with the other. Ask the patient to relax his/her ankle. Bashen and plantar-flex the ankle. Then suddenly dorsi-flex (with moderate manipulation) the ankle and turn the dorsum of the foot outward or inward to remove muscular spasm. Finally, locally and gently Mo, Rou, and Pingtui until the heat produced goes deep.

In the acute stage of sprain (within 24-48 hours after the sprain occurs), conduct light and gentle manipulations and select points not too near to the injured part lest angiorrhexis be worsened around the injury and cause bleeding.

In the restoration stage, perform stronger manipulations to treat hematoma, adhesion, and impaired ankle function. Fumigate and wash with a hot decoction of herbal medicines as needed.

5. Treatment Course: Treatment is given once daily for three days.

6.31 Tarsal Tunnel Syndrome

The tarsal tunnel, located on the medial aspect of the ankle, is a canal enclosed with osseofibrous tissue of the posterior shank and the areolar tissue of the deep sole. Throughout the canal are tendons, blood vessels, and nerves.

Etiology and Pathology:

Sudden increase of movement of the foot or repeated ankle sprain promotes friction of the tendons within the tarsal tunnel. The friction leads to tenosynovitis and thecal cysts, which are responsible for the enlargement of the tendons, blood vessels, and nerves within the tarsal tunnel. Since the tarsal tunnel is an osseofibrous canal that is less flexible than the tendons and blood vessels, it cannot stretch as the content swells. The tunnel portion narrows and the pressure raises within it, resulting in pressure on the posterior tibial nerve.

The tunnel may also be narrowed due to the degeneration and thickness of the ligament, calcaneal spur formation within the tarsal tunnel, or a fracture.

Clinical Manifestations:

Discomfort appearing in the posterior medial malleolus due to walking or standing for long periods of time. In early stages, the discomfort lessens immediately after rest but will appear repeatedly and last longer as the disease becomes severe. More severe manifestations are:

- Numbness in the medial calcaneus and sole
- Dry and bright skin on and around the toes
- Trichomadesis and myophagism of the foot in severe cases
- Exacerbation of a prickling feeling ("pins and needles") when the foot is tapped on the posterior medial malleolus

- Exacerbation of pain in the posterior medial malleolus and the sole when the foot is extremely dorsi-flexed

Treatment:

Better curative effects will be attained when tuina is used to treat tarsal tunnel syndrome due to tenosynovitis and thecal cysts within the tarsal tunnel. Curative effects are lessened or non-existent if tuina is used to treat tarsal tunnel syndrome due to degeneration and thickness of division ligament, calcaneal spur formation within the tarsal tunnel, or fracture. In these instances, operation is suggested.

1. Therapeutic Method: Relax muscles and tendons, promote blood circulation, remove blood stasis, and relieve pain.

2. Manipulation: Yizhichan Tui, Rou, Tanbo, and Ca

3. Point Selection: Yinlingquan (SP 9), Sanyinjiao (SP 6), Taixi (KI 3), Zhaohai (KI 6), and Jinmen (BL 63)

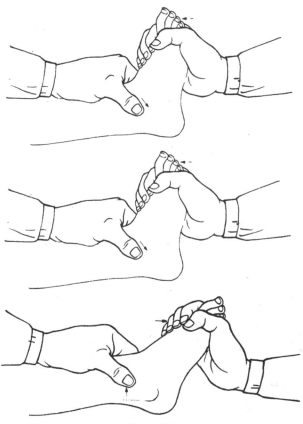

Figure 84

4. Operation:

   a. The patient is supine with his/her affected leg outwardly rotated. DiAn on all the points selected, and Yizhichan Tui on the posteromedial aspect of the shank for five to ten minutes. Yizhichan Tui should be done from top to bottom (with the additional stress on the tarsal tunnel) and vertically along the longitudinal tarsal tunnel.

   b. Tanbo on the part on the tarsal tunnel for three to five minutes.

   c. Ca along the tendon until the heat produced goes deep. Fumigate and wash with a hot decoction of herbal medicines as needed.

5. Treatment Course: Treatment is given once daily for ten days.

6.32 Sprain of Achilles Tendon

There is a special kind of tissue between the Achilles tendon and its superficial deep fascia. It has seven to eight layers. Every pair of layers is connected by connective tissue without adhesion. This tissue functions in lubricating the ankle while it flexes and extends.

Etiology and Pathology:

Acute injury or prolonged repeated strain causes laceration, oozing of blood, or degeneration and necrosis to occur in the tissue between the Achilles tendon and its deep fascia. Subsequently, adhesion forms among the layers and between the layers and the Achilles tendon.

Clinical Manifestations:

The main clinical manifestation is pain in the Achilles tendon.

In the initial stage: Pain usually as soon as movement starts. After movement starts, the pain alleviates, but it may worsen when running or jumping.

In the developmental stage: Pain whenever the Achilles tendon is involved, such as when the patient goes up or down steps or walks. Superficial tenderness, especially evident when the superficial Achilles tendon is twisted, also occurs during this stage.

In the later stage: Degeneration of the tendon, on which there may be palpable geloses. When the tendon is twisted, a cracking sound may be heard. The Achilles tendon loses tenacity and elasticity and is locally thickened into fusiform.

Treatment:

1. Therapeutic Method: Promote blood circulation, remove blood stasis, relax muscles and tendons, and eliminate obstruction from the channels and collaterals.

2. Manipulations: Yizhichan Tui, Nie, Rou, Na, Pingtui, and Yao

3. Point Selection: Taixi (KI 3), Fuliu (KI 7), Chengshan (BL 57), Yangjiao (GB 35), and Ashi point around the Achilles tendon

4. Operation:

   a. The patient is prone with his/her shank, foot, and ankle under a soft cushion. Sit by the affected foot of the patient. Yizhichan Tui to and fro from the Achilles tendon to the popliteal fossa along the gastrocnemius muscle for three to five minutes. Nie and Na—gradually adding pressure—on the Achilles tendon and the gastrocnemius muscle until soreness and distention appear. Then Nie and Na another five to ten times.

   b. Coat the Achilles tendon and the belly of the gastrocnemius muscle with Chinese holly leaf ointment or massage emulsion. Pingtui on it until the heat produced goes deep.

   c. Tui and Rou the Achilles tendon with the thumb for three to five minutes and gently Nie the tissue between the tendon and the fascia; use your thumb and index finger.

   d. Ask the patient to flex his/her knee to 90 and plantar-flex his/her ankle to fully relax his/her Achilles tendon. Hold the patient's dorsum of the foot with one hand and conduct light, quick, gentle NieNa on the posterior aspect of the shank with the other hand. Then Yao the ankle with the hand holding the foot dorsum; gradually widen the amplitude and dorsiflex the ankle.
   After the above manipulations, apply hot compresses, fumigate, and wash with a hot decoction of herbal medicines as needed.

5. Treatment Course: Treatment is given once daily for three days.

6.33 Scapulohumeral Periarthritis

Common in middle-aged and elderly people, scapulohumeral periarthritis usually attacks one shoulder with pain and abnormal function of the shoulder.

Etiology and Pathology:

It is generally thought that this disease is due to insufficient *qi* and blood, irregular nutrition, attack of the shoulder by wind-cold, or trauma and strain. Experimental observation shows that this syndrome is related to the level of sexual hormones.

Clinical Manifestations:
- Soreness, weakness, and limited shoulder movement that appear gradually and usually without any reason
- Pain and/or soreness radiates throughout the shoulder and sometimes radiates to the forearm
- Relieved in the day and so aggravated at night that the patient cannot lie in the affected lateral position.
- Intense pain occurs if the shoulder is touched or the shoulder moves
- Difficult abduction, extension, lifting, adduction, and rotation. When the shoulder is abducted, the patient assumes "pole-carrying" posture (See Figure 85).
- Difficulty in combing his/her hair and dressing and undressing himself/herself.

In the severe cases: The elbow is involved to the extent that the hand cannot reach the shoulder even if the elbow is bent, and atrophy of the deltoid muscle to different degrees occurs.

Treatment:

In the initial stage: Use gentle manipulations locally and repeatedly to remove obstruction from the channels and collaterals, promote blood circulation, relieve pain and strengthen the function of local muscles, tendons, and ligaments.

In the advanced stage: Use more forceful manipulations such as Ban, Bashen, and Yao.

1. Therapeutic Method: Relax muscles and tendons, dredge the collaterals, release adhesion, promote blood circulation, and relieve pain.

2. Manipulations: Yizhichan Tui, DiAn, An, Na, Ban, Bashen, Yao, and Dou

3. Point Selection: Jianneiling, Jianyu (LI 15), Jianliao (SJ 14), Naoshu (SI 10), Tianzong (SI 11), Jianjing (GB 21), Quchi (LI 11), and Hegu (LI 4)

4. Operation:

   a. The patient is supine or sitting. Sit or stand on the affected side of the patient. Yizhichan Tui to and fro on the anterior aspect of the shoulder and the medial aspect of the upper arm for three to five minutes. Then passively abduct, adduct, lift and outwardly rotate the affected arm.

   b. The patient is in a lateral recumbent position with the healthy arm on the bed. Hold the elbow of the affected arm with one hand, and Yizhichan Tui, Rou, or Gun with the other hand on the lateral aspect of the shoulder and the posterior aspect of the armpit. Passively lift and adduct the affected arm.

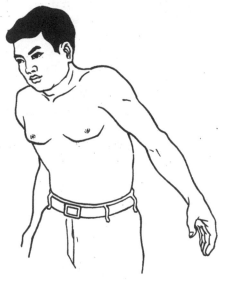

Figure 85

c. The patient is sitting. Na and Nie Jianjing, DiAn, and Rou Tianzong the following points: Naoshu, Jianyu, Jianliao, Jianneiling, Quchi, and Hegu.

d. Stand slightly before the affected arm. Grasp the sore shoulder with one hand, and hold the wrist or support the elbow of the affected arm with your other hand. Rotate the shoulder in small to large circles. Adduct the affected arm by lifting the forearm and flexing the elbow until the patient's hand reaches the healthy shoulder. Repeat the rotation five to ten times. Then conduct NieNa on the disordered shoulder.

e. Stand slightly before the affected side of the patient. Grasp the wrist of the disordered shoulder with one hand, and prop the anterior of the disordered shoulder with your own shoulder. Pull the affected arm back and extend as far as possible with gradually increasing pressure. (See Figure 86). Repeat three to five times.

f. Stand slightly behind the healthy side of the patient; support the healthy shoulder with one hand and grasp the wrist of the affected side with the other. Pull the affected arm to the healthy side via the back of the patient. Do so with gradually increasing pressure and widening range for as long as the patient can tolerate (See Figure 87).

g. Stand to the side of the disordered shoulder of the patient. Hold with both hands the slightly anterior portion of the affected arm's wrist. Lift the affected arm and perform Dou until you lift the arm obliquely upward. Perform these manipulations gently and slowly. While you perform the manipulations, the patient should first drop his/her shoulder and flex his/her elbow, and then stretch and abduct the elbow and lift the arm obliquely upward (See Figure 88).

h. Rotate the disordered shoulder clockwise three times and counterclockwise three times. Cuo with both hands facing each other from the shoulder to the forearm. Repeat three to five times, then Dou the affected arm to end the treatment.

5. Treatment Course: Treatment is given once daily for seven days.

6. Supplements: For better curative effects and earlier recovery, add appropriate shoulder exercises. The exercises should be done diligently and step-by-step. Following are instructions for the exercises. Choose from among the exercises according to the condition of the patient.

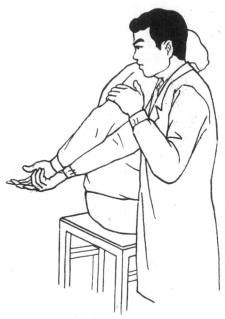

Figure 86

a. Shoulder lifts: Bend the waist, drop both arms, clasp hands together, and swing both arms forward with the amplitude gradually increased.

b. Shoulder abductions: Bend the waist, drop both arms, and swing them to the left and right naturally with the amplitude gradually increased.

c. Backward shoulder extensions: Place your feet shoulder-width apart. Clasp your hands behind your back with the palms facing outward. Using

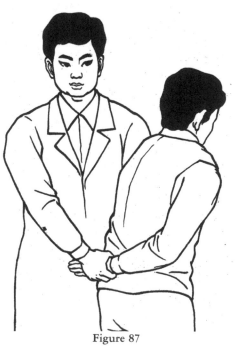

Figure 87

the healthy hand, extend the affected hand as far back as possible; do not bend forward.

d. Shoulder circles: Place your feet shoulder-width apart, stretch both arms out to the side. Circle both arms clockwise and then counterclockwise. Increase the amplitude gradually.

e. Wall-climbing (with hands): Stand in front of a wall. Climb the wall slowly with both hands until they are as high as possible. Repeat several times.

f. Shoulder adduction-abductions: Cross both hands at the back of the neck and adduct and abduct the shoulder as far as possible. Repeat several times.

6.34 Disturbance of Costovertebral Joints

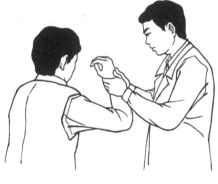

Disturbance (synovial incarceration or mild transposition) of the costovertebral joints is an acute disorder with a sudden onset. It is usually due to improper torsion of the body or violent coughing and sneezing.

Etiology and Pathology:

Synovial incarceration or mild transposition of the costovertebral joints is the cause of this disease.

Clinical Manifestations:

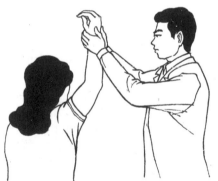

The typical symptom of this disease is sudden pain in one sternocostal area; the pain becomes severe when the patient coughs, sneezes, or takes deep breath. Examination may find out that the patient harbors his/her chest, flexes his/her back,

Figure 88

and takes superficial and short breaths. Examination should also reveal tenderness in the shape of small tracts around the involved costovertebral joints and that traction of the affected arm often causes pain.

Treatment:

Instant results are obtained when this disease is treated with tuina, especially when tuina is applied just after the onset. In cases where treatment is not given right away, inflammatory reaction usually takes place in and around the dislocated joints. If so, recovery will come after several times of treatment.

1. Therapeutic Method: Reduce to stop pain, regulate the *qi* flow, and promote blood circulation.

2. Manipulations: AnRou, Mo, Rou, Bashen, Yao, and Dou

3. Point Selection: Yanglingquan (GB 34) and Chengshan (BL 57)

4. Operation:

   a. Manipulation for relaxation before reduction: The patient is prone. AnRou with the thumb first on Yanglinquan and then on Chengshan for about five minutes to gradually relieve the costodorsal pain and the muscular tension. Then gentle Rou and Mo on the local part for about five minutes to further relieve the pain and muscular spasm.

   b. Manipulation for reduction:

      i. Prop the back to expand the chest: The patient is sitting with his/her hands crossed at the back of the neck. Stand to the back of the patient and hold his/her elbows with both hands. Bend your knee and prop it against the involved costovertebral joints. Using both hands, pull gently backward both of the patient's elbows while pushing your bent knee forward and requesting that the patient take deep breaths. These actions expand the chest. Repeat two to three times. Be sure to pull back and push forward with gentle and slow strength.

      ii. Palm-tapping: The patient is sitting. Stand to the side and slightly behind the patient. Insert your forearm from the front into the patient's armpit and exert force to raise the affected shoulder. Ask the patient to take deep breaths and tap the affected part with the palm root of your other hand. Repeat one to two times.

      iii. Pulled extensions: The patient is sitting on a low stool. Stand before the affected side of the patient. With both hands, hold the fingers of the affected hand with its palm inward. Tightly grasp the hand and inwardly rotate it in a moderately-sized circle from bottom to top. Exert force suddenly to pull the affected arm up when the muscles of the affected arm are relaxed.

c. Ending manipulation: The patient is sitting with the affected arm stretched out to the side. Stand to the lateral-front side of the patient. Hold the patient's wrist and rotate it continuously from the bottom. Circles should be from front to back. Create ten circles, with the patient inhaling when the affected arm is lifted and exhaling when it is dropped. Then grasp the wrist, and pull and shake the affected arm to end the treatment.

5. Treatment Course: Treatment is given one time or until cured.

6.35 Cervical Spondylopathy

Hyperplasia of cervical vertebrae leads to inflammatory stimulation, which compresses the cervical nerve root, spinal cord in the neck, and vertebral artery or sympathetic nerve, causing cervical spondyloapathy. Common in middle-aged and elderly people, the main cause of this disease is degeneration of the intervertebral discs.

Etiology and Pathology:

Injuries to the cervical intervertebral discs, ligaments, and posterior joint capsules due to various acute or chronic trauma decrease the stability of the spine and cause compensatory hyperplasia of cervical vertebrae and compress the nerves and blood vessels.

Hyperplasia of cervical vertebra may occur at the posterior joint, uncinate vertebral joint, and vertebral body. The symptoms of hyperplasia of cervical vertebrae are produced in two ways:

- Direct compression of the nerves and vessels

- Indirect, where local traumatic inflammation and inflammatory congestive edema causes peripheral soft tissues to compress nerves and blood vessels

Clinical Manifestations:

Different sites of hyperplasia display different symptoms.

1. Cervical Spondylopathy of Nerve-root Type: Symptoms due to stimulation or compression of nerve root, which results from retroplasia of the intervertebral facet joints or uncinate vertebral joints are as follows:

- Pain in the neck and shoulder or in the neck and occiput

- Sensory disturbance of the occiput

- Stiffness of the neck

- Radiating pain in the neck, shoulder, and arm(s) accompanied by numbness of the fingers, cold limbs, heavy and weak arms

- Difficulty holding things

- Asymmetrical limitation of cervical movement
- Pain aggravated when extending the neck backward or turning it to the affected side
- Reflex pain and secondary tenderness points on the interior border of the scapula, in the scapular region, or in the shoulder

2. Cervical Spondylopathy of Myeloid Form: Invasion of the protruded intervertebral discs and/or the posterior longitudinal ligament into the vertebral canal causes the spinal cord to compress and patient to display the following symptoms:

- Numbness, soreness, and weakness of the arms, legs, or side(s) of the body
- Quivering neck and trembling arms
- Incomplete spasmodic paralysis marked by limited movement, awkward or staggered gait, dyspnea, hypermyotonia of limbs, tendon hyper-reflexia, weakened or lost superficial reflex, and clonus of the patella and ankle
- Absence of neck ache and dyskinesia (in most cases)
- Incomplete obstruction in a dynamic test of cerebrospinal fluid

3. Cervical Spondylopathy of Vertebral Artery Type: Torsion, spasm, or compression of the artery due to degeneration and hyperplasia of the cervical vertebrae lead to poor blood supply of the vertebral artery. Due to ischemia in the inner ear and brain, symptoms are evoked or worsened by turning or flexing the neck to the side(s). This syndrome is marked by:

- Pain in the neck and shoulder or in the neck and occiput
- Dizziness
- Nausea and vomiting
- Positional vertigo
- Cataplex
- Tinnitus and/or deafness
- Blurred vision.

4. Cervical Spondylopathy of Sympathetic Nerve Type: The symptoms due to the stimulation of the sympathetic nerve are as follows:

- Pain in the occiput
- Heaviness in the head
- Dizziness or migraine

- Palpitation or choking sensation in the chest
- Cold limbs and decreased skin temperature or a feverish sensation in the hands and feet
- Soreness and distention of the extremities
- Absence of radiating pain and numbness sensation in the arm

In some patients, any of the following symptoms may also occur:
- Retrobulbar pain
- Blurred vision and/or photophobia
- Lacrimation
- Rhinorrhea
- A feeling that there is something stuck in one's throat
- Precordialgia
- Facial sweating

5. Cervical Spondylopathy of Anterior Scalene Muscle Type: Protrusions stimulate the fourth and fifth cervical nerve roots and cause spasm of the anterior scalene muscle. The spasmatic muscle compresses the brachial plexus, leading to symptoms similar to cervical spondylopathy of the vertebral artery type.

6. Cervical Spondylopathy of Intervertebral Discs: Degeneration and atrophy of the intervertebral discs stimulate the endings of meningeal branch, causing reflex pain in the neck, scapular region, back, and shoulder. This syndrome exhibits no symptoms.

7. Cervical Spondylpathy of Mixed Type: Two or more types above often mix. When this occurs, the patient exhibits symptoms of the involved types.

Treatment:

Tuina is especially effective when treating cervical spondylopathy. Note: Reduction by turning the cervical vertebrae is not suggested for cervical spondylopathy of the spinal cord type or for patients with hypertension and/or severe arteriosclerosis. When reduction is applied to other types, the operation should be gentle and not violent.

1. Therapeutic Method: Relax muscles and tendons, promote blood circulation, restore and treat injured soft tissues, and conduct reduction.

2. Manipulations: Yizhihan Tui, An, Rou, Na, Bashen, Bashenxuanzhuan, Cuo, Pingtui, Yao, and Dou

3. Point Selection: Fengchi (GB 20), Tianzhu (BL 10), Dazhui (DU 14), Dazhu (BL 11), Jianjing (GB 21), Tianzong (SI 11), Quchi (LI 11), and Waiguan (SJ 5)

4. Operation:

   a. The patient is sitting upright. Stand behind the patient and Yizhichan Tui with your thumb from Fengchi along the sides of the spinous processes of the cervical vertebrae down to Dazhu. Manipulate both sides alternately using a to-and-fro motion. Repeat this five to seven times.

   b. Nie and Na the neck with stress on the pressure point, and gently rotate the neck for two to three minutes.

   c. Perform AnRou with the thumb or the index and middle fingers on Tianzong, Bingfeng (SI 12), Quepen (ST 12), and Jianwaishu (SI 14). Then Na with both hands on Jianjing. Next Tanbo with your index, middle, and ring fingers on the area of the upper one-third of the medial aspect of the upper arm. Finally, AnRou with your thumb on Quchi (LI 11), Shousanli (LI 10), and Waiguan, and then rotate the shoulder in a circle and shake the arm.

   d. Three methods for pulling and extending the neck:

      i. The patient is supine with his/her legs stretched straight and arms flat along the sides of his/her body. Sit directly at the top of the patient's head with your knees against the bed legs. Hold the patient's lower jaw with one hand, and prop the external occipital protuberance with the other hand. Move your waist and the upper body backward to pull the neck with force and to perform Bashen. Shake the cervical vertebrae gently and turn the head left and right softly while Bashen is being done. Repeat this step for two to three minutes. Note: While this is being performed, it is normal sometimes to hear a cracking noise.

      ii. The patient is sitting. Stand behind the patient and put the ulnar sides of both of your forearms on the patient's shoulders. Press downward. Prop the area above Fengchi with both thumbs. Make sure to hold and exert an upward force on the patient's lower jaw with the rest of your fingers and your palms. Press your forearms downward and lift your hands to widen the cervical vertebral spaces. While this is being done, bend the head and neck of the patient forward and backward and turn them left and right.

      iii. The patient is sitting on a low stool. Stand by the affected side of the patient, and with your arm straight, place your hand on the patient's healthy temporo-occipital area and hold the patient's lower jaw. Pull the head slowly upward and, at the same time, turn it left and right. While doing this, use the thumb of your other hand to conduct AnRou on the pressure point of the affected spinous process.

5. Treatment Course: Treatment is given once every two days, ten treatments over 20 days.

6. Supplements: To treat cases with the symptoms of headache and dizziness, also Fenmo (wipe/rub) the forehead and both superciliare arches, DiAn Jingming (BL 1), Yingxing (LI 20), Renzhong (DU 26), and Chengjiang (RN 24). Saosan (sweep/rub) the tempora and the area from the temporo-occipital area to the back of the neck.

Additionally, the patient should do the following neck exercises.

a. Stand with both arms naturally dropped. Relax the whole body. Bend the head and neck slowly forward up to the maximum, and repeat this 20-30 times.

b. Sit or stand. Bend the head and neck laterally and slowly first to the healthy side up to the maximum and then to the affected side to the maximum and repeat this 20-30 times.

iii. Sit or stand. Slowly rotate the head toward the healthy side, then to the back side, the affected side, and the original position. Repeat 20-30 times in this direction, and then reverse directions and repeat 20-30 times.

iv. Sit on a stool with the head in a relaxed upright position. Hold the jaw and occipital region with a traction weight of 3 kg. Hold this position for 30 minutes, and perform traction one to two times daily.

6.36 Stiff Neck

Etiology and Pathology:

Improper pillow height, improper sleeping posture, or exposure of the neck and shoulder to wind during sleep causes myospasm or myofibrositis and results in a stiff neck. It is rarely due to suddenly and improperly turning one's neck or to spasm and sprain from carrying heavy things on one's shoulder.

Clinical Manifestations:

The main manifestations are spasm, stiffness, and pain of sternocleidomastoid muscle and trapezius muscle on one side of the neck. The head is distorted towards the affected side. Movement of the neck is obviously limited. In severe cases, the pain may refer to the head, upper back, and upper arm. The affected area is often tender.

Treatment:

By and large, relief comes after one to two treatments.

1. Therapeutic Method: Relax the muscles and tendons, promote blood circulation, remove obstruction from channels and collaterals, and stop the pain.

2. Manipulations: Yizhichan Tui, An, Rou, Yao, and Na

3. Point Selection: Ashi point, Fengchi (GB 20), Fengfu (DU 16), Jianjing (GB 21), and Tianzong (SI 11)

4. Operation:

   a. The patient is sitting. Stand behind the affected side of the patient. Relax the surrounding muscles by gently applying Yizhichan Tui to the affected side of the neck and shoulder, and, at the same time, support the lower jaw of the patient and push/shake it gently with the other hand.

   b. When the cervical muscles are relaxed and the neck can be turned to larger extent, bend the neck slightly forward and turn it rapidly with the hand supporting the lower jaw to the affected side. This turn should be large in amplitude (five degrees beyond those of the functional position). At the same time, gently push the corresponding spinous processes of the cervical vertebrae towards the normal side with the other hand.

   c. Apply Na to Fengchi, Fengfu, and Jianjing. AnRou to Tianzong, and Pingtui the shoulder until heat is produced.

5. Treatment Course: Treatment is given once daily for three days.

6.37 Disturbance of Lumbar Vertebral Facet Joints

Etiology and Pathology:

This disorder is caused by anatomic disposition of lumbar vertebral facet joints, i.e., dislocation of joints or incarceration of synovium due to an external knock or fall or due to improper movement of the waist.

Clinical Manifestations:

- No prior history of obvious trauma
- Pain that is suddenly felt when the waist twists or bends forward or to the left or right
- Inability to move
- Pain aggravated by coughing and sneezing
- Constant tenderness

- Obviously limited waist movement
- Muscular tension and spasm on the affected side
- Local percussion pain
- No evident tenderness, pain, or restriction of movement in the legs

Treatment:

Once Tuina is used, the cure comes. If treatment is given just after the onset, one treatment is enough.

1. Therapeutic Method: Restore and treat the injured soft tissues, conduct reduction, promote *qi* flow, and stop pain.

2. Manipulations: AnRou, Xieban, and Rou

3. Point Selection: Weizhong (BL 40), Chengshan (BL 57), and the Ashi point in the waist

4. Operation:

   a. Stand or sit to the affected side of the patient in the prone position. Gently AnRou the point of pain with the thumb of one hand, and, at the same time, AnRou Chengshan and Weizhong of the affected side with the thumb of the other hand.

   b. The patient is in the recumbent position with his/her affected leg stretched straight and on the bottom and the other leg flexed on top. Conduct Xieban. Press the patient's hip anterio-inferiorly with one elbow, his/her shoulder postero-inferiorly with your other elbow, and the corresponding spinous process with your thumb. Then exert forces in opposite directions with your elbows to undertake Xieban; a cracking sound may be heard in some cases. Ask the patient to stretch his/her leg with tension, and, while the patient is doing so, pull his/her foot and ankle. Repeat three times or until pain subsides. Finally, gently Rou on the original pain point for two to three minutes.

5. Treatment Course: Treatment is given once. If cure fails to come, continue the treatment until patient is cured.

6.38 Acute Lumbar Sprain

As a pivotal point, the waist controls much of the activity of the body and transmits the weight of the upper body. Loaded with weight and in constant motion, it is easy to injure the waist's muscles.

Etiology and Pathology:

If the loin muscles rotate and pull violently so that the muscles are suddenly injured, acute lumbar sprain occurs. Injury can occur by:

- Extending one's back too far
- Flexing too far forward
- Twisting or bending beyond one's normal range
- Overloading or overexerting the waist
- Assuming continued improper posture
- Falling or some other violent attack

Clinical Manifestations:

In most cases, there is the history of distinct sprain.

1. In severe cases, the patient exhibits the following symptoms:

- Serious loin pain that appears just after the injury
- Limited waist movement
- Difficulty and/or worsened pain when sitting, lying, walking, coughing, sneezing, and breathing deeply.

2. In mild cases:

- Loin pain that is mild just after the injury occurs, but, several hours or days later, is so serious that the waist cannot move.

Treatment:

In the course of treatment, bed rest is suggested so as to avoid re-sprain. For cases with serious pain, hot compress may be added. When undertaking manipulations, select the position in which the patient can feel comfortable, relax his/her limbs, and be sure not to make his/her muscles tense owing to the stress of some position, otherwise, re-sprain may occur.

1. Therapeutic Method: Promote blood circulation to remove blood stasis and eliminate obstruction in the channels and collaterals to stop pain.

2. Manipulations: Rou, Pingtui, Gun, and DiAn

3. Point Selection: Ashi point, Shenshu (BL 23), Weizhong (BL 40), and Chengshan (BL 57)

4. Operation:

   a. The patient is prone. Stand to the affected side of the patient. AnRou the pain point gently with one thumb, and, with the other thumb, apply DiAn to Chengshan on the same side until the lumbar muscles are slightly relaxed. Perform Gun on the lumbar muscles of both sides, gradually increasing the pressure until the pain does not worsen.

   b. Coat the lumbar muscles on both sides with Chinese holly leaf ointment. Pingtui there until the heat produced goes deep into the muscles.

c. The patient is supine with his/her knees and hips flexed. Hold the patient's knees with both hands and gently turn the knees (together) to one side and then the other until patient's waist and hips can move without pain.

5. Treatment Course: Treatment is given once every two days, three treatments over six days.

6.39 Syndrome of the Third Lumbar Vertebral Transverse Process

The third lumbar vertebra is located at the apex of the lumbar vertebrae. Because its transverse process is longer than all the other vertebrae, the third lumbar vertebra acts in a broad range, touches the deep layers of lumbodorsal fasciae often, and bears stronger leverage. As a result, the muscles attached to it tend to be rubbed and pulled, leading to injury.

Etiology and Pathology:

Injury of the muscles and fasciae attached to the third lumbar vertebral transverse process due to overloading or improper twisting of the waist or prolonged repeated lumbar bending will cause tension or spasm of the lumbodorsal muscles. This action stimulates or compresses the lateral branch of the posterior branch of the spinal nerve, and this disease results.

Clinical Manifestations:

- Lumbogluteal pain on one side of the body
- History of lumbar sprain or strain
- Pain radiating along the thigh to the superior of the knee and aggravated when the waist is bent or twisted
- Tenderness at the ends of the third lumbar vertebral transverse process
- Palpable thick, hard, and cordlike mass
- Mild atrophy of lumbar muscles (seen in advanced stages)

Treatment:

In the initial stage of the disease, the manipulations should be gentle. During the course of treatment, the patient should avoid or decrease lumbar extension, flexion, and rotation.

1. Therapeutic Method: Relax muscles and tendons, promote blood circulation to remove blood stasis, and subdue swelling to stop pain.

2. Manipulations: Yizhichan Tui, Ca, Tanbo, and AnRou

3. Point Selection: Ashi point at the ends of the third lumbar vertebral transverse process, Chengshan (BL 57), and Yanglingquan (GB 34)

4. Operation:

   a. The patient is prone. Stand to the patient's affected side. AnRou with your thumb the Chengshan and Yanglinquan points of the affected limb. Use as much pressure as the patient can stand. Then conduct gentle Yizhichan Tui on the affected area where the third lumbar vertebral transverse process is located for three to five minutes.

   b. Perform vertical Tanbo on the cordlike hard mass. Gradually, increase pressure.

   c. Coat the manipulated part with Chinese holly leaf ointment or other lubricating medium, and Ca there until the heat produced goes deep.

   d. Perform Houshenban (backward-extending-pulling) and Jiance Xieban (obliquely-pulling of the normal side).

   e. Use hot compresses on the loins in combination with the manipulations.

5. Treatment Course: Treatment is given once every two days, three treatments over six days.

6.40 Chronic Strain of Lumbar Muscle

Etiology and Pathology:

This disorder is due to prolonged repeated lumbar strain, delayed or maltreated acute injury of lumbar muscle, repeated injury of the lumbar vertebrae, or chronic muscular fibrositis of the lumbus caused by cold and dampness.

Clinical Manifestations:

- History of repeated lumbago manifested as lumbar aching that relapses or becomes severe due to strain
- Pain appearing in the loins when the patient sits or stands for a long time
- Extensive tenderness in the loins
- Palpable tender hard knot with prolonged pain in severe cases
- Muscular spasm
- Lateral curvature of the lumbar vertebrae and pain referring to the legs
- No marked motor impairment in the waist and legs

Treatment:

1. Therapeutic Method: Relax muscles and tendons, activate collaterals, warm up channels, and promote blood circulation.

2. Manipulations: Gun, Rou, DiAn, Ca, and Paiji (pat/hit)

3. Point Selection: Shenshu (BL 23), Mingmen (DU 4), Dachangshu (BL 25), and Weizhong (BL 40)

4. Operation:

   a. The patient is prone. Stand or sit at the side of the patient. Gun over the lumbar muscles of the both sides for about five minutes. Then AnRou with the thumb or the palm root of one hand on the sacrospinal muscles of both sides from top to bottom. Repeat five to ten times with the stress on points Shenshu, Dachangshu, and Zhibian (BL 54). With the thumb of the other hand, DianAn points Weizhong and Chengshan.

   b. Apply massage emulsion or Chinese holly leaf ointment to both sides of the lumbar vertebrae. Ca until the heat produced goes deep.

   c. Paiji the sacrospinal muscles of the lumbodorsal sides.

5. Treatment Course: Treatment is given once daily for seven days.

6.41 Prolapse of Lumbar Intervertebral Disc

Prolapse of the lumbar intervertebral disc is common in young people and is usually due to the prolapse of the fourth and fifth lumbar intervertebral discs and the fifth lumbosacral intervertebral disc.

Etiology and Pathology:

Retrograde affection of aplasia of lumbar intervertebral disc, sudden attack of the loins by external force, or prolonged repeated strain of the waist force the pulpiform nucleus to break through the fibrous ring and protrude backward. This action leads to the compression of the nerve root or the spinal cord. Attack of cold-dampness on the loins causes further injury.

Clinical Manifestations:

1. Lumbocrural pain:

   • History of prolonged recurrent lumbago

   • Pain radiating to one leg (two legs is rare) aggravated by coughing and sneezing

   • Pain or numbness on the lateral or posterior aspect of one shank

- Pain gradually shifting to the loins in some cases
- Tendency to lie on the non-affected side with the affected leg flexed

2. Motor impairment of the loins:

- Discomfort when moving the waist in any direction
- Range of waist movement gradually enlarges with the alleviation of the disease
- Subjective numbness (Subjective numbness is often seen in prolonged cases; the numbness is usually localized on the lateral aspect of the shank and the dorsum, heel, big toe, and/or the sella area).

3. Cold-affected limbs: Coldness and lowered skin temperature in the affected limbs

Treatment

During the course of treatment, the patient should confine himself/herself to bed rest and keep his/her waist warm. When the symptoms and signs are relieved, the patient should do appropriate waist exercises.

1. Therapeutic Method: Reduce, release adhesion, promote the circulation of *qi* and blood, eliminate obstruction in the channels, remove blood stasis, and stop the pain.

2. Manipulations: Qianla, Xieban, Xuanzhuan (rotating) and AnRou

3. Point Selection: Ashi point in the lumbar region, Zhibian (BL 54), Huantiao (GB 30), Yinmen (BL 37), Weizhong (BL 40), Chengshan (BL 57), Yanglingquan (GB 34), and Jiexi (41)

4. Operation:

a. The patient is prone. Stand to the affected side of the patient. AnRou with the thumb on the pressure pain point for two to three minutes. Gradually increase the pressure. At the same time, DiAn-An on the affected side's Weizhong or Chengshan and Yanglingquan points until the lumbar muscles are slightly relaxed. Request that the patient lie on the affected side. Xieban by pressing the deviated process with the thumb. A cracking sound may be heard.

b. The patient is supine. Hold the affected foot and ankle with both hands, and Doula the affected leg three times. AnRou on the spinous process and Weizhong and Chengshan. Rotate and reposition the lumbar vertebrae if necessary to regulate the posterior joints of lumbar vertebrae. Pull the nerve roots and enlarge the nerve root canals and the intervertebral spaces.

Manual counteraction or mechanical traction with a traction table may be conducted with the traction weight 10 kg more than the body weight of the patient. At the same time that traction is being done, press the area around the spinous process so as to reposition the pulpiform nucleus.

5. Treatment Course: Treatment is given once every two days, seven treatments over 14 days.

CHAPTER 7

Tuina for Preventative Healthcare

Self-tuina is performed mainly by self-rubbing and self-pinching and works mainly by activating one's own channel-and-point system. Following is an introduction to the common methods and effects of self-tuina.

7.1 Preventative Self-tuina of the Head, Face, and the Five Sense Organs

Head and Face

1. Effects: Effective in preventing and treating headache, dizziness, insomnia, amnesia, neurosism, and facial paralysis

2. Operation:

   a. Tui on each side of the forehead. Bend both index fingers and, with the interior aspects of the second knuckles, Tui on the midline of the forehead to the midpoint of the anterior hairline. This line runs from Yintang (EX-HN 3) to both Sizhukong (SJ 23) points, Taiyang (EX-S/HE 5), and Touwei (ST 8). Repeat 40-60 times or so (See Figure 89).

   b. Mo on both temples. Put the whorled surfaces of both thumbs tightly on the hairlines around the temples. Repeatedly and with pressure, perform Tui and Mo about 30 times until you feel a sensation of soreness and distension. (See Figure 90).

   c. AnRou on the back of the head. Put the whorled surfaces or the tips of both thumbs tightly on both Fengchi (GB 20) points. With pressure, An ten times. Then, in a rotating pattern, AnRou both Fengchi points, and finally AnRou on Naokong (GB 19) 30 times or until you feel a sensation of soreness and distension (See Figure 91).

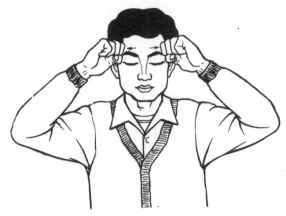

Figure 89

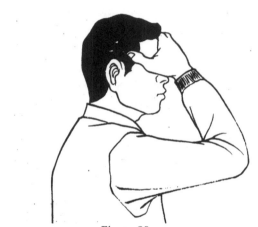

Figure 90

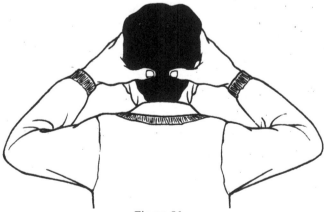

Figure 91

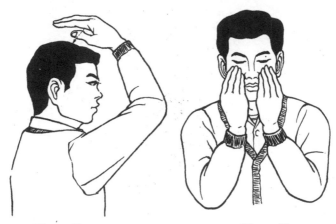

| Figure 92 | Figure 93 |

d. Paiji on the vertex. Sit upright, open your eyes, look straight forward, and clench your teeth. Rhythmically and with your palm, Paiji on the point Xinmen ten times (See Figure 92).

e. Cuo to bathe the cheeks. Rub your the hands against each other until they are warm. Place your palms tightly on the forehead, and Ca with pressure as follows:

  i. down the mandible

  ii. laterally to Jiache (ST 6) along the inferior border of the mandible

  iii. Upward to the midpoint of the forehead via the anterior areas of the areas of the ears and the temples

Repeat 20-30 times or until you feel a sensation of hotness on your face (See Figure 93).

Eyes

1. Effects: Prevention and treatment of various eye diseases such as myopia, blurring of vision, glaucoma and optic atrophy

2. Operation:

a. Rou on Cuanzhu (BL 2). Place the whorled surface of each thumb on each Cuanzhu (BL 2) point (in the depressions proximal to the medial ends of the eyebrows). Gently Rou about 20 times or until your feel a sensation of soreness and distension. Gradually add pressure with each repetition. (See Figure 94).

b. Rou on Jingming (BL 1). Place the whorled surfaces of the thumb and the index finger of the right hand on the Jingming (BL 1) points (in the depression 0.1 *cun* superior to the inner canthus). Press down and squeeze/pinch up repeatedly 20-30 times (See Figure 95).

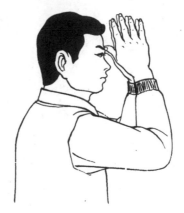

Figure 94

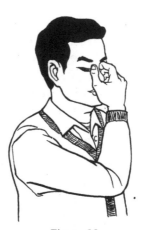

Figure 95

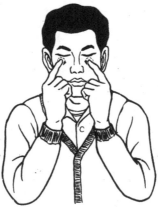

Figure 96

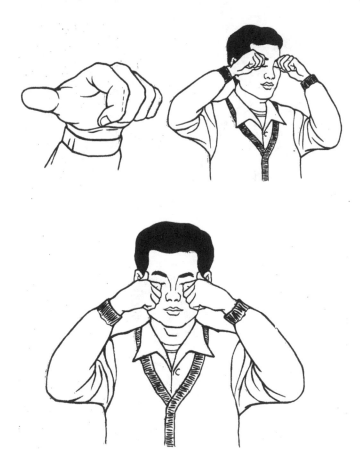

Figure 97

c. AnRou on Sibai (ST 2). Place the whorled surfaces of the index fingers of each hand on the Sibai (ST 2) points (1 *cun* inferior to the midpoint of the lower orbit). AnRou 20 times or until you feel a sensation of soreness and distension (See Figure 96).

d. Gua (scrape) the orbits. Bend the index fingers of both hands, and put the interior aspects of the second knuckles tightly on the internal ends of the upper orbits. Perform Gua from the inside to the outside on the lateral ends of the upper orbits and then on the lower orbits. Repeat the above about 20-30 times (See Figure 97).

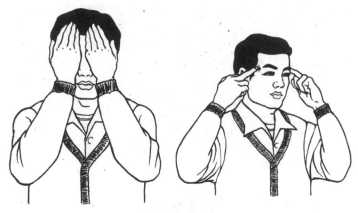

Figure 98   Figure 99

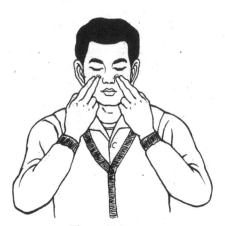

Figure 100

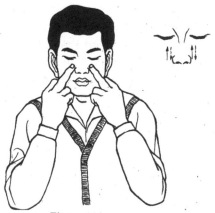

Figure 101

e. Yun (iron) the eyes. Close the eyes lightly (not tightly). Rub your hands until they are warm, and press palms lightly on the eyes to "iron" them for 30 seconds. Then gently Rou the eyes at least ten times (See Figure 98).

f. AnRou on Taiyang (EX-S/HE 5). Place the whorled surfaces of each thumb lightly on the Taiyang (EX-S/HE 5) points. AnRou 30 times or until you feel a sensation of soreness and distension (See Figure 99).

Nose

1. Effects: Effective in preventing and treating the common cold, stuffy and/or running nose, allergic rhinitis, chronic rhinitis, and paranasosinusitis

2. Operation:

a. AnRou on Yingxiang (LI 20). Place the whorled surfaces of both middle fingers on the respective Yingxiang (LI 20) points. With pressure, AnRou 30 times or until your feel a sensation of soreness and distension (See Figure 100).

b. Cuo and Ca on the sides of the nose. Rub the bellies of each index or middle finger to make them warm. Immediately place them on the nasolabial grooves lateral to the wings of your nose. Cuo and Ca up and down 30 times or until heat is produced (See Figure 101).

Ear

1. Effects: Effective in preventing and treating tinnitus, dysacousis, deafness and otitis media

2. Operation:

a. AnRou on the points around the ear. AnRou with the tips of both thumbs or both middle fingers on the respective Ermen (SJ 21), Tinggong (SI 19), Tinghui (GB 2), and Yifeng (SJ 17) points. Press and knead each point 20 times or until your feel a sensation of soreness and distension (See Figure 102).

b. Mo and Ca on the helix. Flex the whorled surface of the thumb and the radial aspect of the index finger like a bow. At the same time, pinch the helixes of both ears. Mo and Ca up and down 20-30 times (See Figure 103).

c. Tanji on the occipital protuberances. Cover both ears with your palms (palm roots in the front and the fingers in the back). Place each of your index fingers on top of each middle finger to conduct Tanji. Your index fingers should slide off the middle ones onto the external occipital protuberances. Repeat 20 times (See Figurs 104).

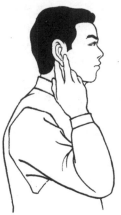

Figure 102

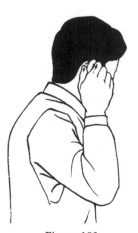

Figure 103

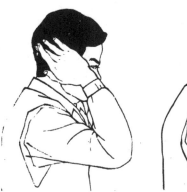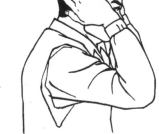

Figure 104

d. Cuo and Ca in front of the ear. Place the radial aspects of both thumbs or the bellies of both index fingers tightly on the anterior areas of the ears. Cuo and Ca up and down. Do this about 30 times or until heat is produced. Then reverse directions and repeat again.

7.2 Preventative Self-tuina of the Extremities

Arms

1. Effects: Effective in preventing and treating scapulohumeral periarthritis, subacromial bursitis, tennis elbow, and carpal tenosynovitis. Also relaxes muscles of the arms, relieves fatigue, improves motor function of the arm joints, and prevents occupational strain.

2. Operation:

   a. AnRou the points (listed below) on each arm—one point at a time, one arm at a time. Use the whorled surface of the left thumb on the right arm and vice versa. Repeat on each point 20 times or until your feel a sensation of soreness, distension, and numbness. The points are: Jianneiling, Jianyu (LI 15) and Jianjing (GB 21) around the shoulder; Quchi (LI 11), Shouanli (LI 10), Chize (LU 57), Quze (PC 3), Shaohai (UT 3), and Xiaohai (SI 8) around the elbow; Waiguan (SJ 5), Neiguan (PC 6), Yangchi (SJ 4), Yangxi (LI 5) and Hegu (LI 4) on the forearm and around the wrist (See Figure 105).

   b. Ca and Tui on the arms. Use the left hand to treat the right arm and vice versa.

      i. With your palm, Ca the anterior, posterior, interior, and lateral aspects of the shoulder, elbow, and wrist. Repeat on each aspect 10-20 times or until heat is produced.

      ii. With the same palm, Ca the channels on the same arm along the following path: From the dorsal carpal cross striation, along the lateral aspect of the arm, straight up to Jianyu at the lateral aspect of the shoulder, via the anterior aspect of the shoulder, along the medial aspect of the arm, and straight down to the intracarpal cross striation. Repeat 30 times or until you feel a warm sensation in the arm (See Figure 106).

      iii. Repeat (i) and (ii) on the other arm.

   c. Ca and Nian on the knuckles.

      i. Ca with the major thenar eminence of left hand on the dorsum of the right hand to warm the intermetacarpal muscles.

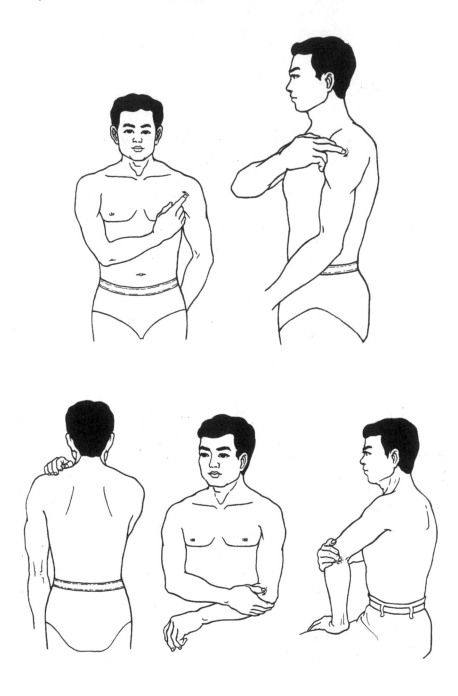

Figure 105

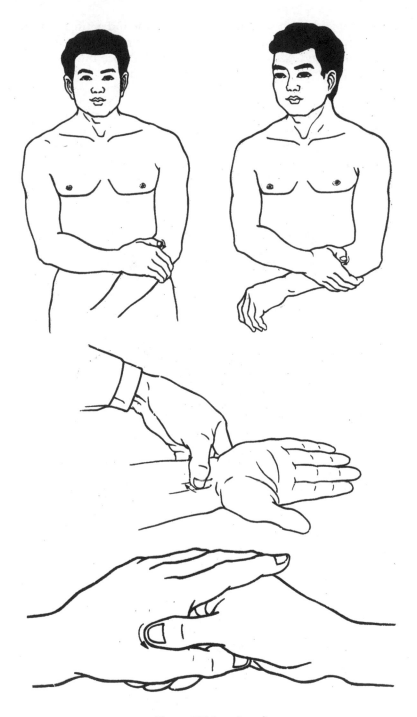

Figure 105 (continued)

     ii. Rou and Nian with the thumb and the index finger of the left hand on the interphalangeal joints of the right hand. Knead and twist one joint after another (See Figure 107).

     iii. Repeat (i) and (ii) on the opposite hand.

Legs

1. Effects: Effective in treating injury of the superior clunial nerves, strain of the gluteal fasciae, swelling and pain in the knee, and systremma and injury of the ankle. Also relaxes the muscles of the legs, relieves fatigue, improves motor function of leg joints, and prevents occupational injuries.

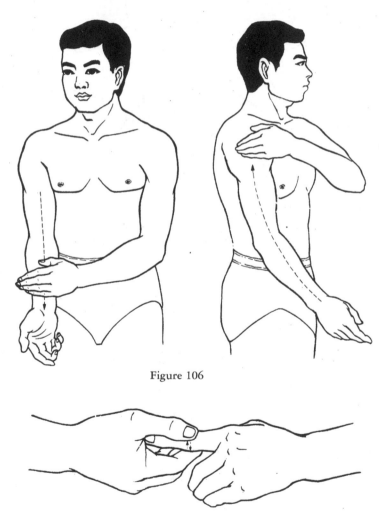

Figure 106

Figure 107

2. Operation:

   a. AnRou on the points over the legs. AnRou with the whorled surface or the tip of the thumb from top to bottom on the following leg points—one leg at a time: Juliao (GB 29), Huantiao (GB 30), Futu (LI 18), Zusanli (ST 36), Yanglingquan (GB 34), Chengshan (BL 57), and Sanyinjiao SP 36). Press and knead each point 20 times or until you feel your *qi* become active there (See Figure 108).

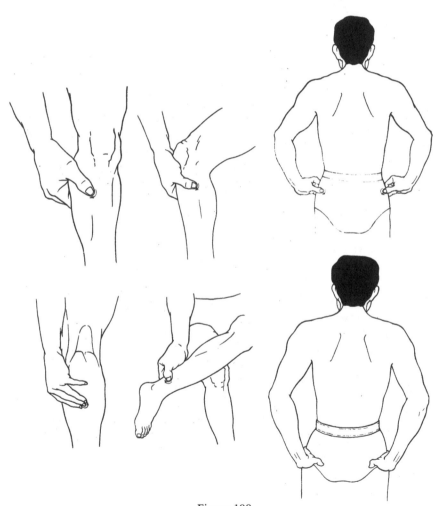

Figure 108

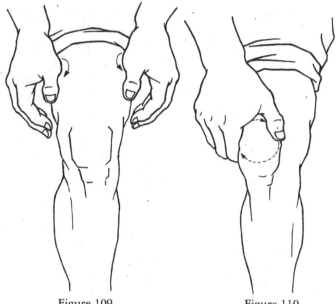

Figure 109   Figure 110

b. AnRou on the thigh. With pressure and using the roots of your palm, AnRou from top to bottom the lateral, medial, and anterior muscles of your thigh. Repeat three to five times until you feel a sensation of soreness and distension (See Figure 109).

c. AnRou on the kneecap. Stretch the legs naturally (with the muscles relaxed). NaNie and AnRou the kneecaps with the belly of the thumb and the radial aspect of the index finger of each hand bent like a bow (See Figure 110).

d. Na on the shank. Gently Ti, Na, Nie, and Rou on the gastrocnemius muscle to the Achilles tendon. Use the thumb and the tips of the index and middle fingers of each hand. Repeat ten times or until you feel a sensation of soreness and distension (See Figure 111).

e. Paiji the legs. Paiji by using the centers of both palms to exert force in opposite directions on the leg from the upper part of the thigh down to the lower part of the shank. Repeat 10-15 times (See Figure 112).

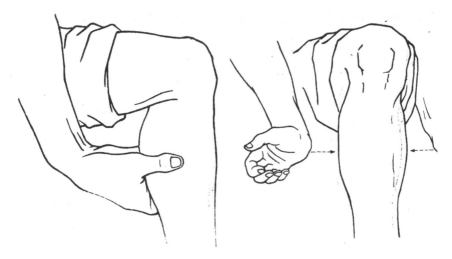

Figure 111   Figure 112

f. Ca on Yongquan (KI 1). Use the hypothenar of one hand to Ca rapidly and with pressure on Yongquan (KI 1)—one foot at a time. Repeat 30 times or until heat is produced. Rub the left foot with the right hand, and vice versa (See Figure 113).

g. Yao on the ankle. Sit upright with the shank of one leg on the knee of the other leg. Hold the superior malleolar portion of the upper shank with one hand and the toes and ball part with the other. Rotate the ankle clockwise and counterclockwise each about 20 times (See Figure 114).

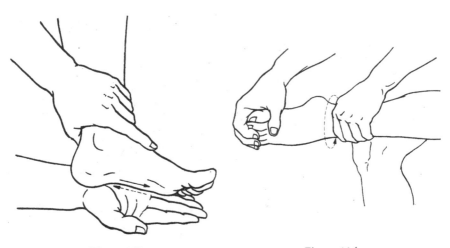

Figure 113   Figure 114

7.3 Preventative Self-tuina of the Chest and Abdomen

Chest

1. Effects: Preventing and treating breathing discomfort or pain, chest pain, a choking sensation in the chest, cough, asthma, disorders of the functional activity of *qi*, and palpitation

2. Operation:

   a. AnRou on the points over the chest and on the intercostal spaces. AnRou with the whorled surface of your middle finger on each of the following points: Danzhong (RN 17), Zhongfu (LU 1), Rugen (ST 18), and Rupang. Repeat 20 times. Then perform AnRou with pressure on the intercostal spaces until each space is pressed and kneaded and you feel a sense of soreness and distension at each space. (See Figure 115).

   b. Na on the muscles of thorax. Apply your thumb firmly to the chest with the index and middle fingers on the lateral part of your underarm. Tina on the anterior axillary fold of the pectoral muscle. Ti and Na alternately and then in combination with slow and gentle Nie and Rou. Repeat the whole routine five times (See Figure 116).

   c. Pai on the chest. Cup the hand and tap the chest along the thoracic median from top to bottom. Repeat ten times and then tap along each of the breast median lines ten times. Be sure not to hold the breath while tapping (See Figure 117).

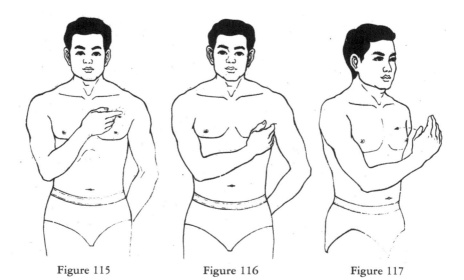

Figure 115   Figure 116   Figure 117

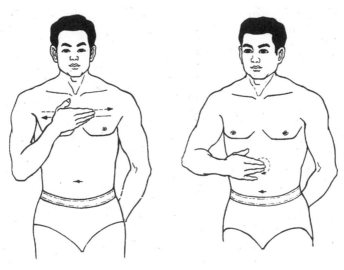

Figure 118   Figure 119

d. Ca on the chest. Place the major thenar eminence of one hand firmly on the surface of the chest and conduct powerful transverse Ca to and fro. Repeat 20 times or until heat is produced (See Figure 118).

Abdomen

1. Effects: Effective in preventing and treating epigastrium discomfort, indigestion, constipation, abdominal pain, irregular menstruation, and impotence

2. Operation:

   a. AnRou on the points over the abdomen. AnRou with the tip of the middle finger, the major thenar eminence, or the palm on each of the following points: Zhongwan (RN 12), Zhangmen (LR 13), Tianshu (ST 25), Qihai (RN 6), Guanyuan (RN 4), and Zhongji (RN 3). Repeat 20-30 times or until you feel the *qi* (See Figures 119 and 120).

   b. Mo on the abdomen. Place your palm around each of the following points (one at a time): Zhongwan (RN 12), Shenque (RN 8), and Guanyuan (RN 4). On each point, conduct circular Mo. Repeat 30-50 times in a clockwise

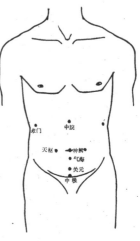

Figure 120

motion and then 30-50 times in counterclockwise motion (See Figure 121).

c. Ca on the lower abdomen. Place the hypothenars of both hands tightly on the Tianshu (ST 25) points (2 *cun* beside the navel). Ca up and down 30 times (See Figure 122).

d. DiAn on Qihai (RN 6), Guanyuan (RN 4), and Zhongji (RN 3). DiAn on Qihai (RN 6), Guanyuan (RN 4), and Zhongji (RN 3), 30-50 times each or so until you feel a sensation of distension and numbness radiating to the external genital organs.

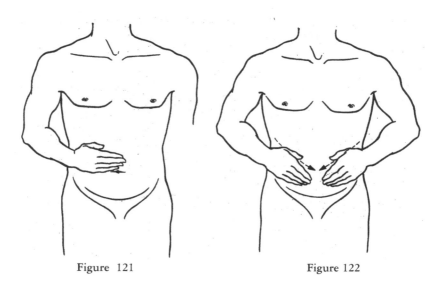

Figure 121   Figure 122

7.4 Preventative Self-tuina of the Neck, Back, and Waist

Neck and Back

1. Effects: Effective in preventing and treating backaches and distension, cervical spondylopathy, stiff neck, cough, asthma, accumulation of phlegm, consumptive disease, choking sensation in the chest, chest pain, palpitation, and angina pectoris.

2. Operation:

a. AnRou on the neck and back.

i. AnRou with the tips of your index, middle, and ring fingers along both sides of Fengchi (GB 20). Proceed via Tianzhu (BL 10) to the root of the neck. Repeat five to ten times.

    ii. AnRou with the tips of the index, middle, and ring
        fingers of one hand along the line from Fengfu (DU 16) to
        Dazhui (DU 14). Press and knead each point about 20-30
        times

    iii. Extend one hand across your back and AnRou with your
        middle finger each of the following points: Dazhui (DU
        14), Dazhu (BL 11), Shenzhu (DU 12), Fengmen (BL 12),
        and Feishu (BL 13). Repeat on each point 30 times or until
        your feel a sense of soreness and distension and then repeat
        the manipulations with your other hand (See Figure 123).

b. Pai on the back. Cup one hand and extend it to the other side
   of the back. Pai on the upper back ten times, and then do the
   same with the other hand (See Figure 124).

c. Mo on Gaohuang (BL 43). Straighten your upper body with
   both arms 90 abducted and the elbows flexed. Rotate both
   shoulders backwards in as large a circle as possible so as to
   stimulate scapulae points such as Gaohuang (See Figure 125).

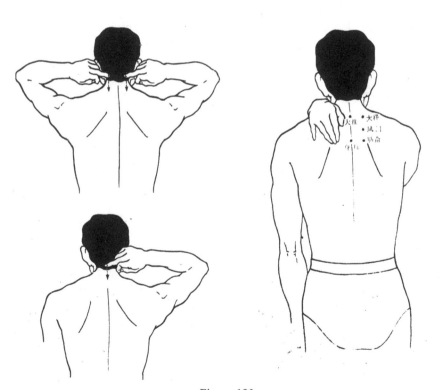

Figure 123

Waist

1. Effects: Effective in preventing and treating aches and pains in the loins, weakness of the waist, insomnia, impotence, frequent urination, lumbar vertebrae proliferation, prolapse of the lumbar intervertebral disc, lumbar muscles strain, irregular menstruation, and diarrhea. Also relaxes the lumbar muscles, relieves fatigue, and improves motor activity of the waist.

2. Operation:

   a. Rou on the points over the loins. AnRou with your knuckles each pair of Shenshu (BL 23), Zhishi (BL 52), and Yaoyan (EX-B7) points. For each pair of points, Repeat AnRou 30 times or until you feel a sensation of soreness and distension (See Figure 126).

   b. Chiuzhen on the lumbar region. Perform tapping, pounding, and vibrating with the ulnar aspects of both fists from top to bottom along the three lines on the lumbar region:

   • The line from Shenshu (BL 23) to Pangguangshu (BL 28)

   • The line from Zhishi (BL 52) via Yaoyan (EX-B7) to Baohuang (BL 53)

   • The line from Mingmen (DU 4) to the lubosaral joint

Repeat Chiuzhen along each line five to ten times (See Figure 127).

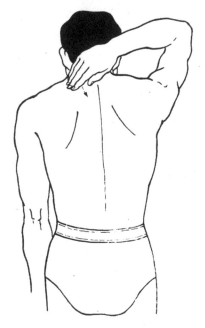

Figure 124

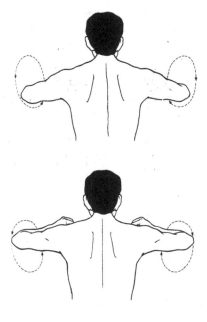

Figure 125

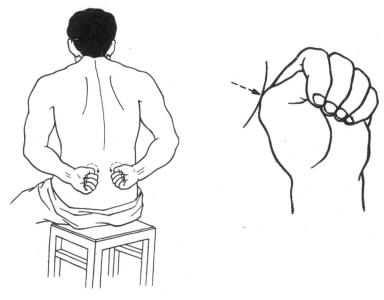

Figure 126

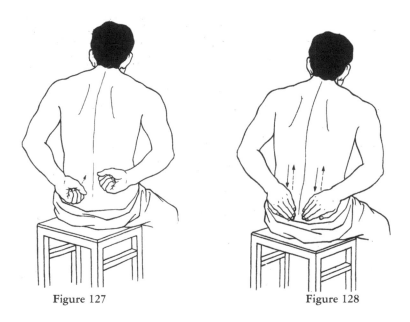

Figure 127   Figure 128

c. Ca on the loins. Press both palm roots hard on the waist, and
   Ca up and down from the second lumbar vertebra to the
   sacro-iliac articulation until heat is produced (See Figure
   128).

Index

Index

BOOKS FROM YMAA

VIDEOS FROM YMAA

more products available from...

YMAA Publication Center, Inc. 楊氏東方文化出版中心

4354 Washington Street Roslindale, MA 02131

1-800-669-8892 • ymaa@aol.com • www.ymaa.com

DEFEND YOURSELF 1 — UNARMED	T010/343
DEFEND YOURSELF 2 — KNIFE	T011/351
EMEI BAGUAZHANG 1	T017/280
EMEI BAGUAZHANG 2	T018/299
EMEI BAGUAZHANG 3	T019/302
EIGHT SIMPLE QIGONG EXERCISES FOR HEALTH 2ND ED.	T005/54X
ESSENCE OF TAIJI QIGONG	T006/238
MUGAI RYU	T050/467
NORTHERN SHAOLIN SWORD — SAN CAI JIAN & ITS APPLICATIONS	T035/051
NORTHERN SHAOLIN SWORD — KUN WU JIAN & ITS APPLICATIONS	T036/06X
NORTHERN SHAOLIN SWORD — QI MEN JIAN & ITS APPLICATIONS	T037/078
QIGONG: 15 MINUTES TO HEALTH	T042/140
SCIENTIFIC FOUNDATION OF CHINESE QIGONG — LECTURE	T029/590
SHAOLIN KUNG FU BASIC TRAINING — 1	T057/0045
SHAOLIN KUNG FU BASIC TRAINING — 2	T058/0053
SHAOLIN LONG FIST KUNG FU — TWELVE TAN TUI	T043/159
SHAOLIN LONG FIST KUNG FU — LIEN BU CHUAN	T002/19X
SHAOLIN LONG FIST KUNG FU — GUNG LI CHUAN	T003/203
SHAOLIN LONG FIST KUNG FU — YI LU MEI FU & ER LU MAI FU	T014/256
SHAOLIN LONG FIST KUNG FU — SHI ZI TANG	T015/264
SHAOLIN LONG FIST KUNG FU — XIAO HU YAN	T025/604
SHAOLIN WHITE CRANE GONG FU — BASIC TRAINING 1	T046/440
SHAOLIN WHITE CRANE GONG FU — BASIC TRAINING 2	T049/459
SHAOLIN WHITE CRANE GONG FU — BASIC TRAINING 3	T074/0185
SIMPLIFIED TAI CHI CHUAN — 24 & 48	T021/329
SUN STYLE TAIJIQUAN	T022/469
TAI CHI CHUAN & APPLICATIONS — 24 & 48	T024/485
TAI CHI FIGHTING SET	T078/0363
TAIJI BALL QIGONG — 1	T054/475
TAIJI BALL QIGONG — 2	T057/483
TAIJI BALL QIGONG — 3	T062/0096
TAIJI BALL QIGONG — 4	T063/010X
TAIJI CHIN NA	T016/408
TAIJI CHIN NA IN DEPTH — 1	T070/0282
TAIJI CHIN NA IN DEPTH — 2	T071/0290
TAIJI CHIN NA IN DEPTH — 3	T072/0304
TAIJI CHIN NA IN DEPTH — 4	T073/0312
TAIJI PUSHING HANDS — 1	T055/505
TAIJI PUSHING HANDS — 2	T058/513
TAIJI PUSHING HANDS — 3	T064/0134
TAIJI PUSHING HANDS — 4	T065/0142
TAIJI SABER	T053/491
TAIJI & SHAOLIN STAFF — FUNDAMENTAL TRAINING — 1	T061/0088
TAIJI & SHAOLIN STAFF — FUNDAMENTAL TRAINING — 2	T076/0347
TAIJI SWORD, CLASSICAL YANG STYLE	T031/817
TAIJI WRESTLING — 1	T079/0371
TAIJI WRESTLING — 2	T080/038X
TAIJI YIN & YANG SYMBOL STICKING HANDS–YANG TAIJI TRAINING	T056/580
TAIJI YIN & YANG SYMBOL STICKING HANDS–YIN TAIJI TRAINING	T067/0177
TAIJIQUAN, CLASSICAL YANG STYLE	T030/752
WHITE CRANE HARD QIGONG	T026/612
WHITE CRANE SOFT QIGONG	T027/620
WILD GOOSE QIGONG	T032/949
WU STYLE TAIJIQUAN	T023/477
XINGYIQUAN — 12 ANIMAL FORM	T020/310
YANG STYLE TAI CHI CHUAN AND ITS APPLICATIONS	T001/181

DVDS FROM YMAA

ANALYSIS OF SHAOLIN CHIN NA	D0231
BAGUAZHANG 1,2, & 3 —EMEI BAGUAZHANG	D0649
CHIN NA IN DEPTH COURSES 1 — 4	D602
CHIN NA IN DEPTH COURSES 5 — 8	D610
CHIN NA IN DEPTH COURSES 9 — 12	D629
EIGHT SIMPLE QIGONG EXERCISES FOR HEALTH	D0037
THE ESSENCE OF TAIJI QIGONG	D0215
QIGONG MASSAGE—FUNDAMENTAL TECHNIQUES FOR HEALTH AND RELAXATION	D0592
SHAOLIN KUNG FU FUNDAMENTAL TRAINING 1&2	D0436
SHAOLIN LONG FIST KUNG FU — BASIC SEQUENCES	D661
SHAOLIN WHITE CRANE GONG FU BASIC TRAINING 1&2	D599
SIMPLIFIED TAI CHI CHUAN	D0630
SUNRISE TAI CHI	D0274
TAI CHI FIGHTING SET—TWO PERSON MATCHING SET	D0657
TAIJI BALL QIGONG COURSES 1&2—16 CIRCLING AND 16 ROTATING PATTERNS	D0517
TAIJI PUSHING HANDS 1&2—YANG STYLE SINGLE AND DOUBLE PUSHING HANDS	D0495
TAIJIQUAN CLASSICAL YANG STYLE	D645
TAIJI SWORD, CLASSICAL YANG STYLE	D0452
WHITE CRANE HARD & SOFT QIGONG	D637

more products available from...

YMAA Publication Center, Inc. 楊氏東方文化出版中心

4354 Washington Street Roslindale, MA 02131
1-800-669-8892 • ymaa@aol.com • www.ymaa.com